Medhumor Medical Publications, LLC

# Laughing Your Way to Passing the Pediatric Boards®

Presents

# Self Assessment Questions & Answers Volume 3

## Clinical Vignettes

By Stu Silverstein, M.D., FAAP

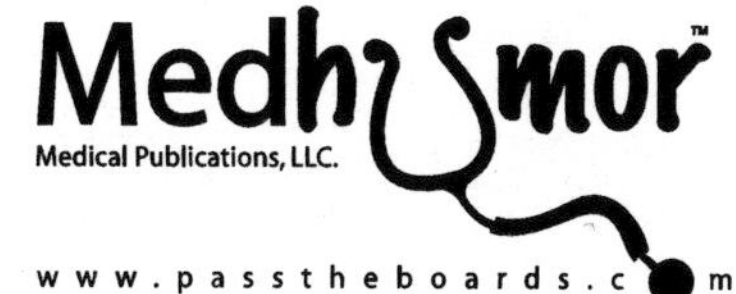


MedHumor Medical Publications, Stamford, Connecticut

**Publisher:** MedHumor Medical Publications, LLC
Stamford, CT.

**Senior Editor:** Andrea Feller, MD, MS, FAAP
Chief Resident,
Preventive Medicine Residency
Program
University of Maryland Medical System

**Design / Copy Editor:** Antoinette D'Amore
A.D. Design
www.addesign-graphics.com

**Cover Designer:** Rachel Mindrup
www.rmindrup.com

**To find more of our titles and information,
please visit us at
www.passtheboards.com**

# About the Author

**Dr. Stu Silverstein** is the founder and CEO of Medhumor Medical Publications, LLC which began with the publication of the critically acclaimed " Laughing your way to Passing the Pediatric Boards"® back in the spring of 2000. Word spread quickly that finally there was a book out there that turned a traditionally daunting process into one that was actually fun and enjoyable. This groundbreaking study guide truly "took the boredom out of board review"® with reports from our readers that they were able to spend half the time studying while retaining twice the material.

The concept of the Laughing your way to Passing the Boards"™ and Medhumor Medical Publications, LLC were conceived by Dr. Silverstein. He brought his years of experience in the field of Standup Comedy and Comedy writing after he realized the critical need for a study guide that spoke the language of colleagues rather than the language of dusty textbooks. His work as a Standup Comedian and Medical Humorist has frequently been featured in several newspapers, radio programs and TV shows, including the New York Times, WCBC newsradio in NY City, as well as World News Tonight with Peter Jennings.

Dr. Silverstein is also a contributing editor for the Resident and Staff Physician annual board review issue and has authored numerous articles on medical humor. He has served on the faculty of the Osler Institute Board Review course and for the UCLA Pediatric Board Review course. He is the co-author of "What about Me? Growing up with a Developmentally Disabled Sibling" written with Dr. Bryna Siegel, professor of Child Psychiatry , UCSF.

Dr. Silverstein is a popular speaker at medical meetings and conferences where he brings his talents as an award winning standup comedian to his "Humor in Medicine .... You must be Joking!!!" presentation. He is also a popular lecturer at residency programs, once again helping residents "take the boredom out of their board review".®

In addition to writing, lecturing, and expanding the scope of Medhumor Medical Publications, LLC., Dr. Silverstein practices pediatric emergency medicine at Our Lady of Mercy Medical Center in the Bronx, an affiliate of New York Medical College.

# Table of Contents

# Introduction

Learning the details required to pass the General Pediatric Exam and Recertification Exam is half the journey. Humor can play an important role in keeping this task fun and in the end can keep you studying longer. We hope that you have found this to be the case with our primary companion text, *Laughing Your Way to Passing the Pediatric Boards*™ 3rd Edition and our *Surfing Your Way to Pediatric Recertification*™. However, studying the text is the equivalent to watching a video on scuba diving. It is now time to put on that wet suit and jump in the water. That's the only way to know if you have the information locked in. Since getting questions wrong can be anxiety provoking, we have integrated the same humorous approach here. Our mission is to "Take the boredom out of board review®."

In response to feedback received from readers we are happy to provide a question and answer book *devoted to case scenarios and vignettes.*

The 3rd volume of our Question and Answer series is compiled of:

**QUESTION SECTION**

Case Scenario

Related multiple choice questions

**ANSWER SECTION**

A step by step analysis of the question

Answers

Explanation

We first provide you with a case scenario followed by a series of question. In the answer section we provide the case scenario in highlighted format with margin notes indicated the significance of the highlighted material.

This illustrates a systematic approach to case scenarios with a proven track record. This is followed by the correct answers and a narrative explanation for these answers.

We are confident that this additional volume of questions and answers will be a useful additional tool that can be used with our main text and other companion titles.

We look forward to hearing from you on how we can improve our materials after you have successfully passed the exam.

The answer sections contain several icon signposts indicating the significance of the highlighted material as follows:

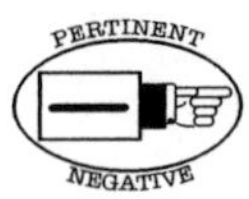


**Pertinent negative**
Pertinent negatives which rule out possibilities in the differential diagnosis

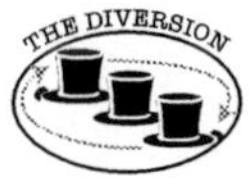


**The Diversion**
Diversions and tricks which might divert you from the correct answers

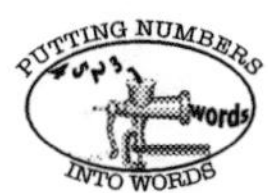


Putting numbers into words
Putting data and other lab values into descriptive adjectives which would be helpful in jogging your memory

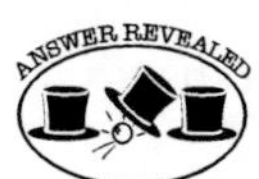


**Answers Revealed**
Indicates text which reveals the answer and is critical to answering the series of questions correctly

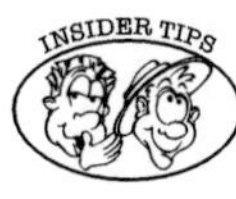


**Insider Tips**
Important tips from those who have been there before

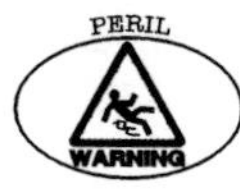


**Peril**
Indicates areas that are notorious for tricking and tripping up exam takers

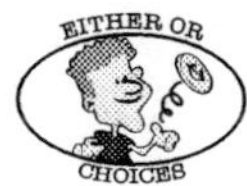


**Either Or**
Indicates similar diagnoses with minute differences and how to distinguish them

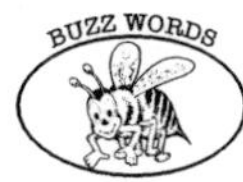


Buzz words
Indicates classic phrases and descriptions which are pathognomonic for a given diagnosis

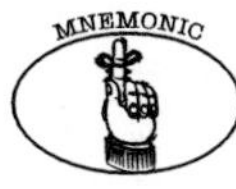


Mnemonic
A mnemonic device for locking specific information into memory

This book will demonstrate how to approach the clinical scenarios presented on the boards systematically so that you can filter out unimportant information and focus on the information that is critical to answering the questions correctly and moving on.

We wish you the best of luck in taking the exam and are confident that you will find our material helpful. We look forward to hearing back from you when you get your test results.

Sincerely,
Medhumor Medical Publications, LLC
www.passtheboards.com

# Questions Section

# Case 1

*(see page 347 for Answers)*

A 9-year-old boy, although very popular with other students, is brought to your office by his parents because of some concerns expressed by his teacher. One example was a book report that was based on the book's illustrations but had no relation to the actual text. He has no difficulty understanding abstract concepts but has a difficult time completing exams that require written explanations. In addition, his handwriting is difficult to decipher. The family denies any extraordinary tension at home and there are no emotional difficulties at school or at home that the parents know about.

## Question 1:

**The child's difficulties are most likely the result of a deficit in:**

A) The ability to focus
B) IQ
C) Phonemic awareness
D) Diet
E) Manual dexterity

## Question 2:

**The intervention most likely to help this child would be:**

A) Methylphenidate
B) Desipramine
C) Fluoxetine hydrochloride
D) Psychotherapy
E) More time to take tests

 

# Case 2

*(see page 349 for Answers)*

An 11-year-old boy in your practice has been having increasing difficulty paying attention in class. In addition to forgetting to take home and complete his homework assignments on time he frequently fidgets in class and talks out of turn. He was diagnosed with ADHD and started on long-acting methylphenidate, which resulted in dramatic improvement in his ability to stay focused at class and at home as evidenced by his turning in his homework assignments on a regular basis.

Over the past few weeks he has been experiencing intermittent facial twitching as well as throat clearing. These increase when he is anxious and at the end of the day when he is most tired.

 

## Question 1:

**What is the most appropriate next step in this child?**

A) Discontinue methylphenidate and implement a behavioral modification program
B) Discontinue methylphenidate and substitute with an SSRI antidepressant
C) Discontinue methylphenidate and substitute with a tricyclic antidepressant
D) Discontinue methylphenidate and substitute with an alpha-2-adrenergic agonist
E) Continue methylphenidate

## Question 2:

**Which of the following medications or class of medications is most likely to cause a movement disorder?**

A) Methylphenidate
B) SSRI antidepressants
C) Tricyclic antidepressants
D) Lithium
E) Dopamine receptor antagonists

 

## Question 3:

**Which of the following statements regarding tic disorders is true?**

A) Tourette syndrome is the most common primary tic disorder
B) The presence of motor tics and coprolalia distinguishes Tourette from other tic disorders
C) Haloperidol is the recommended initial treatment of tics associated with Tourette Syndrome
D) Premonitory urges preceding often represent greater morbidity than the tic itself
E) Voluntary suppression is a useful strategy for managing tics

 

# Case 3

*(see page 353 for Answers)*

You are asked to evaluate a 2-month-old boy who had 2 episodes of vomiting over the past 4 days. The vomiting is non-bilious and "forceful" according to the parents. He is afebrile and his vital signs are stable. He is not feeding well and has been quite irritable. You attempt to feed the baby and notice that the baby arches backward while feeding and you decide to keep the baby in your office to observe while the parents attempt to feed.

His regular pediatrician has diagnosed GERD and started treatment with ranitidine and 2 days ago, when the vomiting progressed, added Reglan® (metoclopramide) which did not improve the symptoms

*(Continued on next page)*

*(Continued from previous page)*

at all. In fact the parents noted similar arching behavior and the "weird movements" you saw in the office. They just thought the baby was tired. His past history is unremarkable and his immunizations are up to date.

A half-hour after trying to feed the baby, he becomes stiff, and clenches his fists with his eyes deviated to the right. He does not respond to tactile stimulation during this episode but there is no color change noted.

After establishing that the baby's vital signs are stable you provide diazepam rectally but the movements continue.

## Question 1:

**Which of the following is the most appropriate *immediate* treatment?**

A) IV diazepam
B) IV lorazepam
C) IV diphenhydramine
D) IM Benztropine
E) PR Promethazine

## Question 2:

**The most likely diagnosis is:**

A) Meningitis
B) Sandifer syndrome
C) Epilepsy
D) Subdural hematoma
E) Acute dystonic reaction

## Question 3:

**Which of the following treatments would be most effective in improving *long-term* outcome?**

A) IV antibiotics
B) Discontinue metoclopramide
C) Start Valproic Acid
D) CT Scan and PICU admission
E) Intubation to protect Airway

 

# Case 4

(see page 357 for Answers)

You are evaluating a 7-year-old girl brought in by her mother who is very alarmed and concerned and asks to speak to you privately while her daughter is having her vital signs taken by your nurse. Over the past week she has noticed that her daughter has been "scratching her privates" more than usual and she has even noticed her doing this in her sleep.

Yesterday she noticed that her daughter was somewhat irritable and had discovered blood on her panties although she did fall on a chair during recess. She also has had bouts of constipation recently. Her past medical history is negative except for a couple of nosebleeds last winter.

*(Continued on next page)*

*(Continued from previous page)*

The parents are married and the patient has a 5-year-old brother and a 10-year-old sister. There have not been any houseguests recently and the mother takes care of the child before and after school. When the mother asked the child she denied that anyone has touched her privates.

On physical examination you note that the hymen is intact with a continuous inner edge, the posterior fourchette does not appear to be friable. However you do note that the labia majora appear to be mildly excoriated with 2 small blood blisters and some dried blood. The labia appear pale and atrophic. The anal opening is within normal limits for age with a small anal fissure, which is barely noticeable.

 

## Question 1:

**The most likely cause of the presenting symptoms in this patient would be:**

A) Lichen Sclerosus
B) Sexual Abuse
C) Vaginal foreign body
D) Straddle injury
E) Physiologic vaginitis

## Question 2:

**The most appropriate management in this patient would be:**

A) Oral Mebendazole
B) Improved hygiene
C) Referral to a sexual abuse clinic
D) High potency steroid cream
E) Report to child protective services

 

# Case 5

*(see page 361 for Answers)*

A 14-year-old girl presents with a one-week history of vague symptoms of malaise, nausea and poor appetitive. Her last menstrual period was a week ago and she had a low-grade fever, which has since resolved.

On physical exam you note several small edematous papules on the hands and face.

Her serum IgM/IgG EBV titers were negative; her Serum beta HCG is negative. Her liver function tests are markedly elevated and her CBC is within normal limits.

You suspect acute Hepatitis B infection.

## Question 1:

**Which of the following would be most helpful in determining if this patient has cleared the virus and is immune?**

A) HBsAg measurement
B) HBeAg measurement
C) Anti-HBs
D) Anti-HBe
E) Anti-HBc

## Question 2:

**Which of the following rises most quickly and is present during acute disease and is a specific reflection of acute disease?**

A) HBsAg measurement
B) Anti-HBc
C) Anti-HBs
D) Anti-HBe
E) IgM Anti-HBc

## Question 3:

**Which combination would indicate an asymptomatic carrier with a low risk of transmitting disease?**

A) HBsAg and Anti-HBe
B) HBsAg and Anti- HBc
C) HBeAg and Anti –HBs
D) HBV DNA and Anti HBc
E) HBV DNA and Anti HBe

# Case 6

(see page 365 for Answers)

You are evaluating a 12-year-old boy who was hit on the left eye by a baseball. There was no loss of consciousness and he has been alert and responsive since with no vomiting or significant headache.
The sclera is injected and he squints when the lights are turned on and he is very uncomfortable.

On ophthalmologic exam you do not see any blood in the anterior chamber of the eye; the eye is equal and reactive with a normal funduscopic examination. Vision screen shows a slight decreased visual acuity in the impacted eye but he can see.

 

## Question 1:

**The most likely diagnosis to explain the presentation would be:**

A) Subdural hematoma
B) Epidural hematoma
C) Traumatic iritis
D) Detached retina
E) Hyphema

## Question 2:

**The most appropriate diagnostic step would be:**

A) Head CT
B) Head MRI
C) Fluorescein staining
D) Measurement of intraocular pressure
E) Slit lamp eye exam

## Question 3:

**The most appropriate treatment would be :**

A) Neurosurgical consult
B) Ophthalmological consult
C) Ketorolac eyedrops and followup
D) Antibiotic eyedrops and followup
E) No medication, followup as needed

# Case 7

*(see page 367 for Answers)*

You grab your chart off the rack and see on the triage note that it is an 8-year-old with abdominal pain and fever. You enter the room to find a child playing and laughing, as he tears the paper off the examining table and drapes it over his parents. You excuse yourself to find the actual room with the patient. His mother jumps up, trailing the examination table paper behind her, and tells you this is the right room.

He is an otherwise healthy very active boy. In fact, he is being treated with methylphenidate for ADHD but only during the week. The family has several pets and the boy plays with them all weekend.

*(Continued on next page)*

*(Continued from previous page)*

Although the boy looks great now, mom says you should see him around midnight when he is doubled over in pain lasting several hours. The next day he is fit as a fiddle. He has had no vomiting or diarrhea.

On Physical examination the boy is tall for his age, vigorous and in better shape than you.

He is afebrile with vital signs stable. There is no rash noted, just several linear scabs on the arm the parents attribute to his horsing around with the pets.

Abdomen- soft, non-tender, with no guarding or rebound tenderness.

You admit the patient and, sure enough, confirm the spiking temperature and the acute episodic abdominal pain.

 

## Question 1:

**The most likely explanation for the abdominal pain would be:**

A) Methylphenidate toxicity
B) Van Münchhausen by proxy
C) Pseudomembranous colitis
D) Microabscesses of the liver
E) Chrons disease

## Question 2:

**The underlying cause of the problem is most likely:**

A) Maternally administered erythromycin
B) Bowel sensitivity to methylphenidate
C) C. Difficile Toxin
D) *Bartonella henselae*
E) Intermittent bowel obstruction

## Question 3:

**The most effective treatment at this point would be:**

A) Bowel rest
B) Corticosteroid enema
C) Azithromycin
D) Metronidazole
E) Switch from methylphenidate to atomoxetine

 

# Case 8

(see page 371 for Answers)

A 15-year-old boy presents with a one-week history of cough and upper respiratory infection symptoms. His right eye has been bothering him and has hurt each time he rubs it, which he admits is a lot of time since he cannot resist the temptation. He presents today because he developed a fever and the right eyelid and surrounding tissue is now red and swollen. All of his immunizations are up to date.

Physical exam confirms a temperature of 101.3 F with marked periorbital swelling, periorbital tenderness and proptosis. His extraocular movements appear to be intact with the exception of upward gaze, which he has difficulty with.

 

## Question 1:

**The most likely diagnosis is:**

A) Periorbital cellulitis
B) Orbital cellulitis
C) Contact dermatitis and secondary infection
D) Dacryocystitis
E) Bacterial conjunctivitis

## Question 2:

**The most likely etiologic organism would be:**

A) *Haemophilus influenza* (non-typeable)
B) *S. epidermidis*
C) *S. pyogenes*
D) *Chlamydia trachomatis*
E) Adenovirus

# Case 9

*(see page 373 for Answers)*

A 7-year-old girl presents with a 7-day history of fever and vomiting. She tells you that she is feeling miserable and has no energy. 4 days ago she developed a rash on her hands and feet which is also present on her back and belly. At that time the family was visiting relatives out of town and the patient was seen in the local emergency room where they got "blood tests" and gave her an IV and some medicines.

You call the ER and confirm that she received IV fluids for dehydration and was given IV Ceftriaxone. Blood cultures are negative.

On physical exam she is ill-appearing with a rash on her trunk, abdomen, feet and hands which can be best described

*(Continued on next page)*

*(Continued from previous page)*

as maculopapular and blanching. You also note some scattered petechiae on her hands and ankles.

Temperature-101.6
HR-130
RR- 45
BP – 80/40

HEENT- dry mucous membranes, EOMI, PERRLA. TM intact, non-injected. Throat – clear
Neck – Supple

Card – S1S2 no murmur
Abdomen – Soft, non-tender, no guarding, decreased bowel sounds.

*(Continued on next page)*

*(Continued from previous page)*

LABS:

CBC- H/H 9/27

WBC- 4.5 82 neutrophils 15

Lymphocytes 3 Monos

Lytes –

Sodium – 125

Bicarb- 19

Glucose – 190

Stool – Culture negative,

positive for occult blood

## Question 1:

**Which of the following is the best test to confirm the suspected diagnosis?**

A) Repeat Blood Culture
B) Monospot
C) EBV IgG/IgM titers
D) Indirect fluorescent antibody testing at the onset of symptoms
E) Indirect fluorescent antibody testing 7-10 days after the onset of illness

## Question 2:

**The most likely diagnosis is:**

A) Kawasaki disease
B) EBV Infectious mononucleosis
C) Rocky Mountain Spotted Fever
D) CMV Infection
E) Meningococcemia

## Question 3:

**The treatment of choice for this patient would be?**

A) Doxycycline IV or PO
B) Await confirmation of indirect antibody fluorescent testing
C) Corticosteroids IV or PO
D) Penicillin VK PO
E) IV Immunoglobulins

# Case 10

(see page 379 for Answers)

You are asked to evaluate a 10-year-old boy who is currently at the 95th%ile for weight and 5th percentile for height.
Up until age 7 the child was at the 75th% ile for both weight and height. He is currently taking no medication and his appetite has not changed-his diet is nutritionally balanced. On physical exam, in addition to marked obesity, you notice several small bruises on his hands and feet.

(Continued on next page)

*(Continued from previous page)*

LABS

CBC

WBC- 19.5

45% neutrophils 45% lymphocytes

10% monocytes

Na/ 139 K/ 2.5 Cl/105 Bicarb/ 25

Glucose/ 75 Bun/ 19 Cre/ 0.4

## Question 1:

**The most likely explanation for the physical findings in this child is:**

A) Prader Willi Syndrome
B) Nutritional obesity
C) Hypothyroid
D) Cushing Syndrome
E) Addison's Disease

## Question 2:

**Which of the following studies would be most appropriate in establishing a diagnosis?**

A) Genetic Karyotyping
B) Nutritional consultation
C) TSH/ T4/ T3
D) Dexamethasone suppression study
E) 17-hydroxyprogesterone level

 

# Case 11

(see page 383 for Answers)

You are called to the nursery to evaluate a full term female baby that according to the nurse "may have ambiguous genitalia". The baby has been feeding well and has been in no distress, except for some difficulty breast-feeding, which is being managed by the lactation counselor. The prenatal course has been unremarkable and the mother denies taking any medication. She was negative for group B strep.

On physical exam the infant is well hydrated, good skin turgor and cap refill < 2 seconds.

*(Continued on next page)*

*(Continued from previous page)*

Examination of the external genitalia reveals a symmetrical swelling of the labia majora, and definite rugae and slight increased pigmentation. There is no clitoromegaly with a normal vaginal and urethral opening. Good urine output is demonstrated with the baby urinating on the blanket you just placed in the bassinet.

LABS

Na/ 139 K/ 4.9 Cl/ 109 Bun/ 14
Cre/ 0.3 Glucose/ 97
CBC- WBC 5.6, normal differential
Platelets – 210 K
H/H 14/45

## Question 1:

**Which of the following would be the most appropriate next step?**

A) Repeat the electrolytes
B) Karyotype
C) Serum 17 Hydroxyprogesterone level
D) IV normal saline bolus and Hydrocortisone
E) Reassurance of nurse and parents in that order

## Question 2:

**Which of the following is the most likely explanation for the physical findings?**

A) Congenital adrenal hyperplasia
B) 21 hydroxylase deficiency
C) Turner syndrome
D) Maternal estrogen
E) Exogenous androgens

 

# Case 12

(see page 387 for Answers)

A 2-year-old presents with a one day history of profuse watery diarrhea, occasionally green in color with no blood noted. Last night he vomited twice and had a tactile temperature with mild abdominal pain. He has not been taking in any PO fluids and it is not clear if he has had any urine output since his stool is too watery.

The parents deny any exposure to toxic substances, and, except for a course of amoxicillin a month ago, he is taking no other medications and he has not eaten any spoiled food. There are 3 children from his daycare who also have diarrhea. His past medical history is unremarkable.

*(Continued on next page)*

*(Continued from previous page)*

On physical exam you note the child to be listless with dry mucous membranes.

Afebrile, HR 150, RR 25, BP 85/60
Cap refill > 3 seconds with extremities cool to touch.

HEENT- TMs intact, no erythema
Mouth – Dry mucous membranes
Throat – Clear, no erythema or exudate
Lungs – Clear
Card – S1S2 No murmur
Neuro – Lethargic, symmetric tone, with DTR 2+ throughout

LAB FINDINGS:

CBC

WBC 11.5
Hgb 12   HCT 36.5   Segs 55%

*(Continued on next page)*

*(Continued from previous page)*

Lymphs 40%   Monocytes 5%
Platelets 220

Lytes
Sodium 136   Potassium 4.5
Bicarb 14   BUN 32   Cre 0.5

UA (cath)

Sp Gravity 1.050   pH 5.2
Glucose negative   Ketones Large
WBC- 2   RBC – 2
Bacteria – negative

## Question 1:

**Which diagnostic study would you order to establish the diagnosis?**

A) Maternal Psych consult
B) Stool for Ova and Parasites
C) Rotavirus antigen testing
D) C. Difficile toxin
E) Stool cultures

## Question 2:

**What is the most appropriate treatment?**

A) Admit for GI consult and Endoscopy
B) Metronidazole PO
C) IV Abilify® (aripiprazole) for mother and hospital CEO
D) IV hydration and overnight admission
E) Attempt PO hydration prior to admission

## Question 3:

**The most effective way to prevent this clinical scenario would be:**

A) Avoid making eye contact with mother and whenever possible the hospital CEO
B) More judicious use of antibiotics in the future
C) Immunization against the etiologic agent
D) Hand washing
E) More effective handling and storage of food products

# Case 13

*(see page 391 for Answers)*

A 21month-old toddler was found by his mother vomiting, coughing and gagging. The mother had just returned from shopping and the child was with his 17 year-old baby-sitter who noted that the toddler did go into the garage 20 minutes earlier for not more than 5 minutes while she ran to the kitchen to turn off the stove, which had been on for quite a while.

The child has no past medical history of any respiratory problems including asthma. There are no household members or recent visitors who are taking any prescription medications.

The toddler is brought to see you in the pediatric ER because the toddler cannot stop coughing and gagging.

*(Continued on next page)*

 

*(Continued from previous page)*

On physical exam the child is afebrile with a HR 125, BP 90/50, $SaO_2$ 92% on room air. RR 45, Lungs are clear to auscultation, no wheeze or rales. He is tachypneic and coughing.

## Question 1:

**The most likely cause of the coughing and gagging in this toddler would be:**

A) Exacerbation of asthma from dust
B) Foreign body aspiration
C) Carbon Monoxide exposure
D) Hydrocarbon ingestion
E) Organophosphate Ingestion

## Question 2:

**What is the most appropriate *next* step in treatment?**

A) Chest X-ray
B) Give supplemental $O_2$
C) Syrup of ipecac
D) Albuterol nebulizer treatment
E) Arrange for transfer to a facility with a hyperbaric chamber

## Question 3:

**The *most* appropriate management of this patient would be:**

A) ICU admission with continuous albuterol nebulizer treatments
B) CXR and discharge from ED if CXR is negative
C) CXR and observation with repeat CXR in 6 hours
D) IV atropine
E) Discharge on home nebulizer and oral steroids

# Case 14

(see page 395 for Answers)

An 18-year-old girl presents with a 3-day history of abdominal pain and vomiting, which is worsening. She is afebrile and has had no diarrhea.

She has had intermittent abdominal pain over the past 6 months diagnosed as irritable bowel syndrome. She is non-icteric. The pain is dull at the moment but can be sharp and she sometimes experiences back pain as well.

She is not sexually active and is not taking birth control pills. Denies drinking alcohol or any illicit drug use.

Past history is significant for a diagnosis of bipolar depression at age 15 for which she is being treated

*(Continued on next page)*

*(Continued from previous page)*

with valproic acid as a mood stabilizer. Her levels were last checked 10 days ago and were within therapeutic range.

On physical examination she is non-icteric. Her vital signs are stable. On abdominal exam her pain is mostly epigastric and left upper quadrant with no guarding or rebound tenderness. There is no hepatosplenomegaly and bowel sounds are normal.

Her mouth is dry and the remainder of the exam is unremarkable.

LABORATORY FINDINGS

WBC – 14.5 H/H 15/45

Platelets – 238 K

*(Continued on next page)*

*(Continued from previous page)*

Sodium/ 140 Potassium/ 4.0
Chloride/ 105 Bicarb/22
Glucose/ 145 Bun/9
Creatinine/0.2

Aspartate aminotransferase/189
Alanine aminotransferase/338
Alkaline phosphatase/324

Bilirubin-

Total 2.5 Direct/ 1.4

Total Protein/7.4 Albumin/4.2

Calcium/9.2

ABG 7.45/36/68

Oxygen Saturation – 98 % on Room Air

Abdominal Ultrasound – multiple gallstones and no focal pancreatic lesions

 

## Question 1:

**Which of the following studies would be most useful in establishing the correct diagnosis at this stage?**

A) Serum Amylase and Lipase
B) CT Scan with Oral Contrast
C) CT Scan with IV contrast
D) CT Scan with oral and IV contrast
E) Endoscopy

## Question 2:

**Which of the following should be included in the acute management of this patient?**

A) IV antibiotics
B) Meperidine
C) Morphine
D) Surgical removal of the gallstones
E) Endoscopic retrograde cholangiopancreatography

## Question 3:

**This condition is associated with each of the following EXCEPT:**

A) Hypercalcemia
B) Hypocalcemia
C) Hyperglycemia
D) Hypoglycemia
E) Hyperlipidemia

 

# Case 15

(see page 401 for Answers)

A 14-year-old boy is brought in by EMS after being discovered in the garage by his parents obtunded after one episode of emesis. His mother reported that he had complained earlier of blurred vision.

His father had been in the garage the previous night winterizing the car and doing other work on the engine. Several chemicals were left in one-liter soda bottles on the work bench, as noted by the paramedics on the scene. The patient also enjoys working on cars and has frequently worked with his dad. He is also an honor student.

On Physical examination:
No odor of alcohol was noted on the breath and has had no history of drinking alcohol.

*(Continued on next page)*

*(Continued from previous page)*

Vital Signs:

Afebrile, Respiratory Rate – 36 per minute, HR – 160, and BP 140/85

The lungs were clear. Cardiac – 2+ pulses, cap refill < 2 seconds, normal sinus rhythm with no murmurs. Abdominal exam – soft, non-tender, no guarding or rebound tenderness. No organomegaly. Neurological exam- The patient appears to be lethargic and groggy. 2+ DTR throughout with symmetrical tone and strength.

LABORATORY FINDINGS –
Sodium 146 mEq/L,
Potassium 4.2 mEq/L,
Chloride 107 mEq/L,
Bicarbonate 14 mEq/L,
Serum urea nitrogen 12 mg/dL,
Creatinine 0.9 mg/dL,

*(Continued on next page)*

*(Continued from previous page)*

Blood glucose 148 mg/dL,
Total serum calcium 10 mg/dL,
Phosphorus 5.1 mg/dL,
Magnesium 2.8 mg/dL.

Urinalysis was normal, with the exception of the presence of calcium oxalate crystals.

Arterial blood gas:
pH 7.12,
PaO2 71 mm Hg,
PCO2 30 mm Hg.

## Question 1:

**The most likely cause of the child's condition would be toxic ingestion of:**

A) Methanol
B) Ethylene Glycol
C) Organophosphates
D) Ethanol
E) Hydrocarbon

## Question 2:

**The most important initial step in managing this patient would be:**

A) Ethanol as an antidote
B) IV atropine
C) Head CT
D) IV Normal Saline bolus
E) Intubation

## Question 3:

**The long-term complications of concern in this patient would be:**

A) Blindness
B) Severe chemical pneumonitis
C) Renal failure
D) Cerebral Hemorrhage
E) Sudden death

# Case 16

(see page 405 for Answers)

You are asked to see a 22-month-old girl because of developmental delay and odd features that your family practice colleague cannot quite identify. The child's physical growth was on target for the first year but then trailed off. The girl is not walking yet and has not spoken any complete words.

The child has had an extraordinary number of respiratory infections. You agree that the child does have some odd features including a rather large head and a face that is a bit too harsh, especially for a female; as well as an enlarged tongue and corneal clouding. Exam is also significant for hepatomegaly and a 3/6 systolic ejection murmur.

## Question 1:

**The most appropriate initial step in identifying the diagnosis in this child would be:**

A) Karyotyping
B) Measure serum mucolipid levels
C) Measure serum glycoprotein levels
D) Measure urine mucopolysaccharide (GAG) levels
E) Head CT

## Question 2:

**The most likely diagnosis for this child would be:**

A) Fragile X syndrome
B) Tay Sachs disease
C) Hunter syndrome
D) Hurlers syndrome
E) Niemann Pick disease

## Question 3:

**Which of the following additional findings are associated with children with this diagnosis?**

A) Hearing loss
B) Testicular enlargement
C) Micropenis
D) Normal intelligence
E) Retinal cherry red spot

# Case 17

*(see page 409 for Answers)*

You are evaluating a 16-year-old girl who for the past week has had a "bad cold and cough". The cold has gotten "a little better" but the cough has remained the same and her chest also feels tight and her chest hurts. The pain is intermittent but seems to get worse when she lies down. In addition, she has experienced RUQ tenderness, back pain and some nausea and vomiting.

Her past medical history is unremarkable and other than oral contraceptive pills she is not taking and has never been prescribed any medications.

*(Continued on next page)*

*(Continued from previous page)*

**Physical Exam:**

Temp – 99.1
Respiratory Rate- 25
HR- 101

She is in no apparent distress at rest
HEENT – throat clear, TMs intact, non-injected
Neck – supple, no palpable lymph nodes
Lungs – Clear, no wheeze, rales or rhonchi
Card – S1 S2, normal sinus rhythm, 2+ pulses throughout with cap refill < 2 seconds
Abdomen- soft, mild RUQ tenderness with no guarding or rebound, no hepatosplenomegaly
Back – mild right-sided flank pain.

*(Continued on next page)*

*(Continued from previous page)*

**Laboratory studies –**

Venous Doppler ultrasound / Legs – Negative

## Question 1:

**Which of the following studies are likely to reveal the cause of this patient's symptoms?**

A) Renal Ultrasound
B) Abdominal ultrasound
C) Chest X-ray
D) Chest CT
E) Abdominal CT

## Question 2:

**This workup is most likely to reveal which of the following diagnoses?**

A) Pyelonephritis
B) Renal Stone with hydronephrosis
C) Pneumonitis
D) Pulmonary embolus
E) Acute appendicitis

## Question 3:

**Which of the following would be the most appropriate treatment?**

A) Trimethoprim –Sulfamethoxazole
B) IV hydration and pain management
C) Surgical consult
D) Albuterol aerosol and PO antibiotics
E) Heparin and warfarin

 

# Case 18

(see page 415 for Answers)

You are evaluating a 12-year-old girl who has just recovered from a recent viral illness and has been having difficulty walking over the past few days. You note weakness in her legs with deep tendon reflexes of 1+. Upper extremity strength is normal with deep tendon reflexes 2+. There is no point tenderness over the vertebral spine and MRI earlier this week was negative.

## Question 1:

**The most pressing concern in this patient is risk for:**

A) Cardiac arrest
B) Uncal herniation
C) Respiratory arrest
D) Airway obstruction
E) Permanent paralysis

## Question 2:

**Which of the following would be most useful in establishing the correct diagnosis would be?**

A) Muscle Biopsy
B) Lumbar puncture
C) Head CT
D) Abdominal CT
E) EKG

## Question 3:

**The most likely diagnosis in this patient is:**

A) Duchenne's muscular dystrophy
B) Becker's muscular dystrophy
C) Transverse myelitis
D) Ruptured vertebral disc
E) Guillain Barré disease

 

# Case 19

*(see page 417 for Answers)*

You are called to the nursery at 6:30 AM just prior to change of shift to evaluate a newborn with a concerning rash. The baby was born full-term with an uneventful prenatal course and normal spontaneous vaginal delivery.

On Physical exam you note a skin eruption on the infant's face and scalp which is a violaceous-dusky color with skin atrophy in the middle of papular scaly eruptions. There is no hepatosplenomegaly on physical exam. Lungs are clear to auscultation and heart sounds are normal, S1S2 with no murmur.

**CBC-**
WBC- 9.5
H/H – 36/12
Platelet Count 125
EKG- Unremarkable

## Question 1:

**Which of the following would be most helpful in establishing the etiology of the findings in this infant?**

A) Skin biopsy
B) Blood Culture
C) Liver Function Tests
D) Tzanck smear
E) Serum anti-Ro (ssA) level

## Question 2:

**What would be the most appropriate management and treatment?**

A) IV Antibiotics
B) Admission and IV acyclovir
C) Head CT
D) Discharge and judicious use of sun block
E) Indirect sunlight

## Question 3:

**Which two medications are BOTH appropriate for the treatment of CMV infection**

A) Zapemall and Foscarnet
B) Acyclovir and Ribavirin
C) Amantadine and Acyclovir
D) Ganciclovir and Acyclovir
E) Ganciclovir and Foscarnet

# Case 20

(see page 421 for Answers)

A 6-year-old with a one-week history of vomiting presents to your office. He is afebrile, with no diarrhea. He was seen in the emergency room last night while the parents were driving home from a camping trip. He was prescribed promethazine suppositories and told to followup with you. He has had no episodes of vomiting last night and has remained afebrile.

The parents are concerned because he appears to be weak and he is unsteady and needs some assistance standing up. He also claims that you have two heads and only one is talking.

On physical examination the child exhibits unsteady gait with diplopia.

*(Continued on next page)*

*(Continued from previous page)*

Other than that his neurological examination is normal with symmetrical tone and strength and 2+ DTR throughout. His abdomen is soft with no guarding, rebound or tenderness. There is no hepatosplenomegaly. He is pale with dry mucous membranes.

## Question 1:

**Which of the following is most likely to reveal the underlying problem?**

A) Serum electrolytes
B) Diphendydramine
C) Metronidazole
D) Normal Saline Bolus 20 cc/kg
E) Head CT

## Question 2:

**Which of the following is the most likely cause of the patient's presentation?**

A) Hyponatremic dehydration
B) Hypernatremic dehydration
C) Dystonic Reaction
D) *Giardia Lamblia*
E) Arterio-venous malformation

# Case 21

(see page 425 for Answers)

A 3-month-old presents with diarrhea and is irritable with poor feeding. There is no reported history of vomiting. The stools have large "curds" in them and are yellow-brown in color.

The mother is feeding the baby modified formula in powdered form.

The child has been very irritable and mom was told by a neighbor that the child is probably hungry and she needs to make the formula stronger, which the mother says she has done.

PHYSICAL EXAM –

Lethargic, ill appearing
Temperature 101.2 F
HR-180
RR- 70
Weight 5 Kg

*(Continued on next page)*

*(Continued from previous page)*

Skin – pale, mottled with dry mucous membranes.

Lungs - clear

Card – normal with weak distal pulses

Abdomen- distended, no mass, no guarding

Neuro – hyperactive, deep tendon reflexes

Skin – doughy, and redundant abdominal skin is noted.

LABS

H/H 11/33

WBC 21 with a normal differential

Sodium- 169

Potassium – 4.9

Bicarb – 15

*(Continued on next page)*

 

*(Continued from previous page)*

Bun – 25

Cre- 0.6

Urinalysis unremarkable

You diagnose hypernatremic dehydration due to increased solute loss secondary to concentrated formula.

 

## Question 1:

**Which of the following is true regarding hypernatremic dehydration?**

A) Clinical signs may be masked due to fluid shifts from intracellular to extracellular space
B) Clinical signs may be masked due to fluid shifts from extracellular to intracellular space
C) Sensorium usually deteriorates early on
D) Hypernatremia is defined as a serum sodium concentration greater than 150mEq/L
E) A urine concentration > 150 mOsm/kg suggests a diagnosis of diabetes insipidus

## Question 2:

**Which of the following is true regarding the treatment goals of hypernatremic dehydration?**

A) The serum sodium should be gradually reduced over 18 hours
B) The serum sodium should be gradually reduced over 24hours
C) Rapid lowering of the serum sodium level can result in shifting water out of the brain cells
D) Rapid lowering of the serum sodium level can result in shifting of sodium into the brain cells
E) Hypernatremic dehydration can result in subarachnoid and subdural hemorrhaging

# Case 22

(see page 429 for Answers)

You are evaluating a 12-year-old boy with a known history of asthma. Today he received several treatments with aerosolized albuterol and continues to wheeze. On physical examination he is afebrile and has diffuse wheezing on expiration. The chest x-ray reveals some consolidation with significant volume loss on the left side.

## Question 1:

**The most likely explanation for the child's exacerbation is:**

A) Atelectasis
B) Tension pneumothorax
C) Acute bacterial pneumonia
D) Acute viral pneumonia
E) Aspergillosis

## Question 2:

**The most important step in treating this patient would be:**

A) Change in chronic management
B) Immediately start antibiotics
C) Antipyretics and respiratory therapy
D) Oral steroids
E) IV Voriconazole

# Case 23

*(see page 431 for Answers)*

A 16 year-old girl with Type 1 diabetes since the age of 10 presents with severe abdominal pain and dry mouth. The smell of nail polish remover permeates the room so you look around but nobody has nail polish or appears to have recently removed the nail polish. The patient and parents insist that they follow a strict sliding scale regimen and are compliant.

Her ABG reveals a pH of 7.29, serum glucose is 710 and her urine is positive for glucose and ketones.

Her physical exam is negative except for mild chest pain and abdominal pain with no guarding or rebound.

## Question 1:

**The most important initial step in managing this patient would be:**

A) Glycosylated hemoglobin level
B) SQ Insulin based on her sliding scale
C) 1/2 NS with 20 mEq KCL/ 20 mEq K Phos. @ 1.5 maintenance
D) NS Bolus 20 cc/KG
E) CT Scan with Contrast

## Question 2:

**The patient is now stabilized. Which statement regarding management over the next few hours is most appropriate?**

A) Begin insulin drip 1 unit/Kg /hour
B) Begin insulin drip 0.1 units/Kg/hour
C) Adjust SQ insulin due to illness
D) Add 5% glucose when serum glucose levels are below 125 mg/dL
E) Reduce Serum glucose to below 150 within 2 hours of admission
F) Have security search everyone's bags to find out who used your bottle of nail polish remover without permission

 

## Question 3:

**Which of the following is true regarding the long-term management of children with Type 1 diabetes?**

A) Low glycosylated hemoglobin closely correlates with number of reported episodes of severe hypoglycemia
B) Despite close correlation between severe hypoglycemia episodes and low glycosylated hemoglobin, the discomfort is worth the long term gain
C) There is no correlation between low glycosylated hemoglobin levels and episodes of severe hypoglycemia
D) There is a negative correlation between low glycosylated hemoglobin and episodes of severe hypoglycemia
E) Glycosylated hemoglobin levels are not as significant in children as adults

 

# Case 24

*(see page 433 for Answers)*

You are evaluating a 3-year-old girl with URI symptoms. During your examination you note that the patient has a lower than usual hairline with some facial asymmetry. The patient is developmentally delayed and the parents note that the child has a mild hearing deficit. Her neck has a decreased range of motion and appears to be shorter in proportion to the rest of the body with a webbed appearance. Cervical spine x-ray reveals fusion of cervical vertebrae 2 and 3.

## Question 1:

**Which of the following is the most likely diagnosis?**

A) Turner syndrome
B) Sprengel Syndrome
C) Posterior Fossa Tumor
D) Klippel Feil Syndrome
E) Trisomy 21

## Question 2:

**Which of the following associations is most likely to be seen in this patient?**

A) Cervical muscle spasm
B) Horseshoe kidney
C) Delayed puberty
D) Atanto-axial instability
E) Cleft palate

# Case 25

*(see page 435 for Answers)*

You are presented with a 6-week-old infant who, up until this point, has been a well-appearing, thriving infant. The baby was initially icteric on day 2 of life, which resolved without any intervention and the mother has continued to breast-feed. The infant was the product of a full-term gestation delivered by normal spontaneous vaginal delivery with Apgars of 9 and 9. There is no family history of liver disease.

On physical examination, the baby is noted to be well-nourished and in the 75th %ile for height, weight and head circumference. There are no obvious dysmorphic features. The baby is icteric including the sclerae and the rest of the exam is unremarkable.

*(Continued on next page)*

*(Continued from previous page)*

The serum indirect and direct bilirubin is 10.1/8.2

## Question 1:

**The most likely explanation for the baby becoming icteric again would be:**

A) Breast–milk jaundice
B) Alagille syndrome
C) Neonatal hepatitis
D) Biliary atresia
E) TORCH infection

## Question 2:

**The most appropriate next step in diagnosing the underlying cause would be:**

A) Hepatitis B core and surface antigen titers
B) Liver biopsy
C) Abdominal ultrasound
D) Serology for TORCH infection
E) Trial of formula feeding

## Question 3:

**Which of the following would be helpful in making the *definitive* diagnosis?**

A) Hepatitis B core and surface antigen titers
B) Liver biopsy
C) Abdominal ultrasound
D) Serology for TORCH infection
E) Trial of formula feeding

# Case 26

(see page 439 for Answers)

A 4-1/2 month old infant is brought to your office because the infant has not been himself, is lethargic, vomited twice last night and had a fever of 102.3 which was brought down to 100.1 with acetaminophen.
He has had not diarrhea. He has been around other children with a viral gastroenteritis.

Physical examination shows a temperature of 101.5, respiratory rate of 25 and heart rate of 130 beats per minute. The baby seems to be very lethargic and difficult to console.

HEENT – TM, red with decreased mobility and bulging on the right side. EOMI, PERRLA AF is full

Neck – supple, no meningismus

*(Continued on next page)*

*(Continued from previous page)*

Lungs – clear

Card – S1 S2 no murmur, pulses 2+ throughout.

Abdomen – soft

Skin – no rashes noted

Neuro – symmetrical tone and strength

LABS

CBC

WBC – 19.5 60 % neutrophils, 34% bands, 6% Lymphocytes

H/H 9/36

*(Continued on next page)*

*(Continued from previous page)*

**Lumbar Puncture:**

Gram Stain –negative

Latex agglutination – negative

Glucose – 20

Protein- 80

Urinalysis – negative

 

## Question 1:

**The most likely explanation for the infant's symptoms is:**

A) Viral gastroenteritis
B) Right otitis media
C) Viral syndrome
D) Intracranial mass
E) Bacterial meningitis

## Question 2:

**The most appropriate initial management would consist of:**

A) Oral rehydration and antipyretics
B) IV hydration and antipyretics
C) Oral amoxicillin
D) IV Cefotaxime
E) IV Vancomycin and Cefotaxime

 

# Case 27

(see page 443 for Answers)

You are asked to evaluate a 6-week-old infant who a presents with inspiratory stridor and intercostal retractions.
On physical examination you note that the child's cry is weak and the infant occasionally becomes cyanotic.
The stridor has been present since birth.

 

## Question 1:

**Which of the following is the most likely explanation for the infant's condition?**

A) Bilateral vocal cord paralysis
B) Unilateral vocal cord paralysis
C) Laryngomalacia
D) Tracheomalacia
E) Subglottic stenosis

## Question 2:

**Which of the following would best confirm diagnosis:**

A) Microlaryngoscopy
B) Flexible bronchoscopy
C) Rigid bronchoscopy
D) Flexible upper airway endoscopy
E) Chest CT

# Case 28

*(see page 447 for Answers)*

You are called in by your obstetric colleague to evaluate a new rash on a woman who is at 39 weeks gestation. Of course, your colleagues call you in to evaluate rashes rather than the dermatologist because of your availability and much more favorable rates.

You stroke your chin with your double gloved hand and look at the centrally umbilicated vesicular lesions concentrated on the trunk and their erythematous base; with several other similar lesions on the extremities, some of which are erythematous pruritic macules.

 

## Question 1:

**You place a third glove on your hands and continue to stroke your beardless chin, then you reveal the following correct diagnosis:**

A) Disseminated Herpes Simplex
B) Herpes Zoster (Shingles)
C) Chickenpox
D) Scabies
E) Macula-papular-eczematous pruritic non-specific dermatitis

## Question 2:

**The most appropriate management in this case would be:**

A) Dependent on the timing of the delivery
B) Elective C-section
C) Elimite(R) and Scabies protocol
D) IV Acyclovir
E) To note that you will need to review a scraping under the microscope after submitting your CPT coded bill

## Question 3:

**The woman delivers the baby precipitously while the obstetrician ponders your answer. The most appropriate treatment at this point would be:**

A) IM Varicella –zoster immunoglobulin to the baby
B) IM Varicella – zoster immunoglobulin to the mother
C) Administer the live varicella vaccine now
D) Culture the mother's lesions and start the baby on IV acyclovir
E) Reassurance only

# Case 29

*(see page 449 for Answers)*

You are caring for a boy in your practice that repeatedly injures his right knee. Each injury results in a massive effusion and pain. After several negative orthopedic consults and MRIs you come across a pediatrician triple-boarded in pediatric EM, hematology and sports medicine who correctly diagnoses the problem as Hemophilia A. There is no family history of hemophilia.

## Question 1:

**Which of the following statements are true regarding Hemophilia A?**

A) Female carriers usually present with metrorrhagia at the onset of menses
B) Female carriers never have clinical signs of hemophilia
C) Less than 5% of children with hemophilia are a result of new mutations
D) Factor activity level less than 30% results in frequent episodes of hemarthroses with mild trauma
E) Female carriers can present with bleeding during pregnancy or surgery

## Question 2:

**Which of the following is the most common initial presentation of hemophilia?**

A) The vast majority of males are diagnosed at the time of circumcision
B) Soft tissue bleeding when they start crawling
C) Multiple episodes of hemarthroses in large joint depending on activity
D) Multiples episodes of hemarthroses of hands when using utensils and large toys
E) The presentation is largely variable depending on the environment

## Question 3:

**The most appropriate management of bleeding episodes for patients with Hemophilia A would be:**

A) Factor 9 replacement at home
B) Factor 9 replacement in a hospital setting
C) Factor 8 replacement at home
D) Factor 8 replacement in the hospital setting
E) FFP infusion in the hospital setting

 

# Case 30

(see page 453 for Answers)

A 16-week-old afebrile infant presents with a runny nose and cough for the past 2 to 3 days. The baby has been breast fed with some supplementation. Breast-feeding has gone well. She was delivered by normal spontaneous vaginal delivery at full term with no complications. The prenatal course was unremarkable except for one time when the mother accidentally ate a piece mahi mahi maki sushi in Hawaii but spit most of it out on the floor several feet away on a surfer's booties. Group B strep cultures were negative and no intrapartum antibiotics were given.

Physical examination shows that the infant has intercostal retractions and

*(Continued on next page)*

*(Continued from previous page)*

bilateral rales, with a respiratory rate of 52 breaths/min and a heart rate of 128 beats/min. Oxygen saturations are 96%. CXR shows diffuse infiltrates

## Question 1:

**How did the infant most likely acquire this infection?**

A) In your office during the 2-week visit
B) Transplacentally
C) During the birth process
D) By droplet infection
E) By airborne infection

## Question 2:

**The most appropriate treatment in this case would be:**

A) Albuterol via nebulizer with close followup
B) Oral prednisone, albuterol via nebulizer and hospital admission
C) Oral Prednisone with close followup
D) Oral Azithromycin (Zithromax®)
E) HIV testing and Trimethoprim-Sulfamethoxazole

# Case 31

*(see page 457 for Answers)*

A 14-year-old afebrile girl presents with acute onset of right lower quadrant tenderness with severe nausea and vomiting. The pain is sharp in nature and radiates to the back. She has not had dysuria, urgency, or diarrhea. The pain has been intermittent over the past 24 hours sometimes lasting 1-2 hours and then resolving spontaneously. Her last menstrual period was 3 weeks ago and she is sexually active but "always uses protection."

On physical exam she is in considerable pain with vital signs within normal limits. Her abdomen is soft but tender with no guarding or rebound tenderness.

*(Continued on next page)*

 

*(Continued from previous page)*

The abdominal pain is increased over the right lower quadrant.

Bowel sounds are present. Bimanual exam reveals right sided adnexal tenderness with no increased cervical motion tenderness

CBC – WBC- 9.5 with a normal differential

Na/ 139 K / 4.0 Cl/ 105 Glucose/ 95 Bun/ 15 Cre/ 0.3 Bicarb/ 24

Urinalysis – negative except for 20 RBC

Urine HCG – Negative

 

## Question 1:

**Which of the following would be most helpful in establishing a diagnosis?**

A) Abdominal CT
B) Cervical Cultures
C) Serum Quantitative HCG
D) IVP
E) Abdomen x-ray flat and upright

## Question 2:

**The most likely diagnosis is:**

A) Intrauterine pregnancy
B) Ectopic pregnancy
C) Renal stone
D) Ovarian Torsion
E) Small bowel obstruction

## Question 3:

**Which of the following interventions would be indicated after establishing the diagnosis?**

A) Salpingo-oophorectomy
B) Laparoscopic exploration
C) Methotrexate
D) IV hydration, analgesia and alkalinization of the urine
E) General Surgery consultation

 

# Case 32

*(see page 461 for Answers)*

An 8-year-old boy presents with a patchy distribution of hair loss over the past 8 weeks. On physical exam you note 2 areas of hair loss in the frontal region of the scalp that are complete, with the exposed skin appearing smooth. There are no broken hairs noted and no erythema. The rest of the physical exam is unremarkable except for nail pitting.

 

## Question 1:

**The most likely diagnosis is:**

A) Alopecia neurotica
B) Trichotillomania
C) Alopecia areata
D) Tinea capitis
E) Tension alopecia

## Question 2:

**The most appropriate treatment would be:**

A) Topical antibiotics
B) Oral antibiotics
C) Topical antifungal cream
D) Oral Antifungal
E) Reassurance

 

# Case 33

(see page 463 for Answers)

An 18-year-old female returns from winter break complaining of palpitations and difficulty sleeping as well as weight loss and decreased appetite. On physical examination you notice a tremor in both of her hands and her eyes seem to be more pronounced than you would like.
She is also unable to tolerate heat and sleeps with the windows opened even when it is below freezing outside.
There is a symmetrical non-tender mass over her anterior neck.
She was a straight "A" student in high school and has been struggling to get C's in college. She is taking no medications and her urine tox screen and pregnancy test are both negative.

 

## Question 1:

**Which of the following would be the most appropriate next step?**

A) Ask her if she is comfortable with her weight
B) Refer her for a psychiatric evaluation
C) Serum T3, T4, and TSH levels
D) Abdominal CT
E) Head CT

## Question 2:

**Which of the following is the most likely diagnosis?**

A) Hashimoto's disease
B) Bipolar mood disorder
C) Addison's disease
D) Pheochromocytoma
E) Graves disease

## Question 3:

**The most appropriate treatment for this patient would be:**

A) Mood stabilizers
B) Hydrocortisone
C) Alpha blockade followed by surgery
D) Beta blockade followed by surgery
E) Thyroid ablation

 

# Case 34

(see page 465 for Answers)

A 12-year-old girl presents because of a severe cough that has kept her up at night and out of school for the past 3 days. She had the flu including high fever, vomiting and diarrhea and cough. All but the cough symptoms have resolved. The mother notes that she has had "chronic bronchitis" since she was a child. In the past, Azithromycin has worked wonders. Fortunately she had an extra pack in one of the shoeboxes in her shoe closet but it has not helped this time. She would like you to treat the bronchitis this time.

## Question 1:

**The most likely explanation for the persistent coughing would be:**

A) Outdated medication
B) Aspergillosis
C) Psychogenic cough
D) Bronchospasm
E) Mycoplasma pneumonia

## Question 2:

**The most appropriate treatment for this patient would be:**

A) Azithromycin
B) Amoxicillin
C) Psychotherapy
D) Albuterol via metered dose inhaler
E) Oral prednisone for 5 days

## Question 3:

**The patient returns a month later with a similar history only this time on physical exam you notice a slight expiratory wheeze and more discomfort. The most appropriate additional treatment at this point would be:**

A) Amoxicillin-Clavulanic acid
B) Levalbuterol via metered dose inhaler
C) More Psychotherapy
D) Oral Montelukast daily
E) Oral prednisone for 5 days

# Case 35

(see page 467 for Answers)

A 14-year-old girl complains of recurrent headaches, which are throbbing and pulsating in nature and felt most severely behind her right eye. She is a competitive cross country skier and the headaches are most severe when she is training the hardest or otherwise exerting herself physically. She experiences no muscle cramping with the headaches. The headaches are usually accompanied by waves of nausea and vomiting. She is meticulous with rehydrating during training consistent with training protocol confirmed by her trainer. The only relief for her headaches is lying down and sleeping in a quiet room with the lights dimmed. She has avoided seeking medical attention because of fears she will be told to quit skiing and

*(Continued on next page)*

*(Continued from previous page)*

with a college scholarship in the wings this is not an option. She has also taken no medications fearing this would disqualify her from Olympic trials.

She is popular with friends and has maintained her grades despite the increasing frequency of her headaches. You obtain a urine HCG, which is negative and her last menstrual period was 2 weeks ago and has been regular.

PHYSICAL EXAM:

General – well nourished female with weight and height in the 60th percentile for age
HEENT – no evidence of papilledema, EOMI, PERRLA
SMR (Tanner) – 3

*(Continued on next page)*

*(Continued from previous page)*

Lungs – clear

Card – S1, S2 no murmur, normal sinus rhythm, cap refill less than 2 seconds

Abd- soft, non-tender

 

## Question 1:

**The most appropriate next step in establishing a diagnostic explanation for this patient's symptoms would be:**

A) Urine Tox screen
B) Psychiatric evaluation for an eating disorder
C) Head CT
D) Psychological counseling and analgesics
E) Addition of salt pills and potassium supplements for fluid replacement

## Question 2:

**Which of the following diagnoses best explains the patient's presentation?**

A) Performance enhancing steroids
B) Bulimia nervosa
C) Migraine headaches
D) Tension headaches
E) Salt and Potassium depletion during training

## Question 3:

**The most appropriate intervention for this patient would be:**

A) Postpone training for 6 months
B) Referral to a nutritionist
C) Ibuprofen and close followup
D) Psychological counseling
E) Corrective lenses

 

# Case 36

*(see page 471 for Answers)*

A 12-year-old girl appears at your office on a Friday at 5:05 PM (for her 3:30 PM one Wednesday) in the cold and dark of December. Her mother tells you that the girl has been limping for a couple of weeks because of severe left-sided knee pain.
Her past medical history is negative except for continued weight gain despite several attempts to lose weight with the help of a nutritionist.
They live in a wooded area and she has not traveled recently.

She has been afebrile, and does not recall being hit in the knee or leg.
She is taking no medications and has not had any recent viral illnesses.
She has difficulty moving her leg inward.

 

## Question 1:

**The most definitive diagnostic study would be:**

A) AP and lateral X-ray Left Knee
B) Anteroposterior and frog lateral x-rays of the pelvis
C) Bone Scan
D) CBC, Blood Culture, ESR
E) Lyme titers

## Question 2:

**Given the late hour and that the workup will be done in the emergency department, you impress the pediatric emergency department staff by telling them that the most likely diagnosis is:**

A) She twisted the leg trying to be on time for the appointment Wednesday
B) Arthritis secondary to Lyme disease
C) Septic arthritis of the knee
D) Aseptic necrosis of the hip
E) Slipped capital femoral epiphysis left hip

## Question 3:

**The most appropriate treatment would be:**

A) Amoxicillin for 6 weeks
B) Hospital admission for IV antibiotics
C) Surgical correction
D) IV antibiotics, knee immobilizer and crutches
E) Limited physical activity for 6 weeks and close followup

# Case 37

(see page 473 for Answers)

You are evaluating an afebrile 15-year-old girl with severe abdominal pain and vomiting but no diarrhea. The pain has occurred over the past 2 days and radiates to her back. She has remained afebrile and has not changed her diet nor has she traveled out of the U.S. recently. The pain is severe and intermittent and has interfered with her sleep although she can sleep once the pain subsides. On physical examination the pain is primarily in the right upper quadrant. There is no significant family history of any GI disease.

 

## Question 1:

**Which of the following studies would be most appropriate initial step in establishing the correct diagnosis?**

A) Serum HCG
B) Urinalysis
C) Abdominal CT with IV contrast
D) Serum amylase and lipase
E) Abdominal ultrasound

## Question 2:

**The most likely diagnosis in this patient would be?**

A) Cholecystitis
B) Cholelithiasis
C) Primary pancreatitis
D) Pregnancy
E) Pyelonephritis

## Question 3:

**What is the most appropriate next step in managing this patient once the correct diagnosis is established?**

A) Transvaginal ultrasound
B) ERCP
C) IV antibiotics and discharge when stable
D) Cholecystectomy
E) Analgesics and close followup

# Case 38

(see page 475 for Answers)

A 3-year-old girl presents with a fever of 100.2°F and severe ear pain. It is a Saturday morning and you are covering for their regular pediatrician, Dr. Treatemall. According to the parents, "this happens all the time," with this being the 3rd episode in 6 weeks. The child's aunt, who up until now was quietly sending text messages in the corner, blurts out "Dr. Treatemall always gives us the pink medicine and sometimes the white fruity one except for that one time he gave us the yellow tutti-fruity ones which were the only samples he had left in his pocket!"

On Physical exam, the child is afebrile with stable vital signs. Respiratory rate is 32 and unlabored.

*(Continued on next page)*

*(Continued from previous page)*

The child is alert, with some discomfort, nasal congestion, and slight cough. Lungs on auscultation are clear, no rales, wheeze or rhonchi. Cardiac exam reveals S1 S2, normal sinus rhythm, pulses 2+ throughout with cap refill < 2 seconds.

Her tympanic membranes are red, with positive movement on insufflation. The tympanogram does show a peaked curve.

## Question 1:

**The medical student working with you asks which diagnostic studies would be most appropriate in this patient?**

A) Referral to an immunologist due to the frequency of the illnesses
B) RSV antigen immunofluorescence
C) Myringotomy for positive identification and treatment
D) CBC CXR, and Blood Culture
E) No diagnostic studies are indicated at this point

## Question 2:

**What would be the most appropriate treatment?**

A) Antihistamines and decongestants
B) Acetaminophen
C) Azithromycin (Zithromax®)
D) Amoxicillin/potassium clavulanate (Augmentin ®)
E) Ask the aunt to text message Dr. Treatemall to see if he has any more tutti-fruity antibiotico-booty left

 

# Case 39

*(see page 479 for Answers)*

You are evaluating a 7-year-old boy who has had bouts of excruciating abdominal pain for well over a year. The parents are besides themselves and have had their son evaluated by a nutritionist, herbologist, homeopathic doctor and even a pediatric gastroenterologist at the university medical center. Despite a "boatload of tests" done by all of these consultants, the pain continues. The pain is worse in September and seems to get better during the summer and during winter and spring break.

He has had no weight loss and is at the 60th percentile for weight and height. He has experienced intermittent headaches with the belly pain and some nausea but no diarrhea or constipation. Stool is heme negative and has been normal in size and color.

 

## Question 1:

**The most likely explanation of this child's abdominal pain is:**

A) Crohn's disease
B) Ulcerative colitis
C) Pituitary tumor
D) Functional recurrent abdominal pain
E) Celiac Sprue

## Question 2:

**The most appropriate next step in managing this patient is:**

A) Small bowel biopsy
B) Colonoscopy
C) Head CT
D) Barium Enema
E) Reassurance and counseling

## Question 3:

**The long-term prognosis for this patient is:**

A) Variable depending on frequency of exacerbations
B) Excellent with colectomy
C) 5 year survival is excellent with radiation
D) Excellent with gluten free diet
E) Symptoms will continue into adulthood in up to 50% of patients

# Case 40

*(see page 481 for Answers)*

A 2-year-old presents with a 4-day history of cough and respiratory distress and chest tightness, which has gotten progressively worse. Except for 2 episodes of post tussive emesis he has had no vomiting or diarrhea. The parents are careful to keep choking hazards out of reach and do not believe he ingested or aspirated any foreign bodies. The father smokes but always in a different room or outside.

His past history is significant for 3 episodes of lobar pneumonia, twice requiring hospitalization. You look up his medical records from his previous admissions and note that both times he had pneumonia involving the right lower lobe.

*(Continued on next page)*

*(Continued from previous page)*

He was born at 37 weeks gestation and was large for gestational age. The delivery was traumatic with Apgars of 4 at one minute and 9 at 5 minutes. He was in the NICU for 4 days and required some supplemental oxygen. There was decreased movement of his right arm diagnosed as Erb's palsy but with some physical therapy his range of motion is almost fully recovered.

On physical exam he is in moderate distress breathing at 75 breaths / minute, heart rate is 165, with an oxygen saturation of 90% in room air. He has a temperature of 101.2.

*(Continued on next page)*

 

*(Continued from previous page)*

His lungs are clear but there are significant subcostal and intercostal retractions with nasal flaring. There are decreased breath sounds on the right side.

CXR – right lower lobe infiltrate as well as elevation of the right hemidiaphragm

## Question 1:

**Which of the following studies would be most helpful in establishing the correct diagnosis?**

A) Real time Fluoroscopy
B) RSV antigen testing
C) Pulmonary function testing
D) Inspiratory/Expiratory chest film
E) Chest CT

## Question 2:

**The most appropriate short-term intervention would be:**

A) Inpatient management and isolation
B) IV ceftriaxone
C) Racemic Epinephrine aerosol as needed
D) Subcutaneous terbutaline
E) Continuous albuterol aerosol

## Question 3:

**The most effective long-term intervention would be:**

A) Buy the father a smoking jacket and smoking room in another county
B) Home nebulizer
C) Oral Solu-Medrol for 5 days
D) Allergy testing
E) Referral to Pediatric Surgery

# Case 41

*(see page 485 for Answers)*

You are evaluating a 7-month-old infant who has become increasingly jaundiced over the past few weeks. With the exception of mild hyperbilirubinemia during the initial postnatal days, the baby has not been jaundiced at all. The mother's blood type is A+ and the baby is O negative. The baby has been not been gaining weight adequately since 2 months of age. On physical examination you note wide spaced eyes and a smaller than usual mandible.

On physical exam the baby is icteric. Lungs are clear and the cardiac exam is normal except for a grade 3/6 murmur.

The total and direct bilirubin is 7.6/5.5

 

## Question 1:

**The most likely explanation for the hyperbilirubinemia is:**

A) Gilbert syndrome
B) Alagille Syndrome
C) Neonatal hepatitis
D) Pierre Robin Syndrome
E) Fetal Alcohol syndrome

## Question 2:

**Each of the following additional findings would be expected *except for*:**

A) Marked hepatomegaly
B) Vertebral anomalies
C) Pulmonic stenosis
D) Hyperlipidemia
E) Cutaneous xanthomas

## Question 3:

**The approximate life expectancy for this baby for the first decade of life would be:**

A) Full life expectancy with episodic hyperbilirubinemia
B) Full life expectancy with appropriate dietary control
C) Full life expectancy with liver transplantation
D) 70% with liver transplantation
E) 70% with no intervention

 

# Case 42

*(see page 489 for Answers)*

A 2-year-old boy is brought to your office because of persistent high fever despite being given ibuprofen every 8 hours as suggested on the bottle. He was seen in the emergency room when the fever started one week ago and was given amoxicillin for an ear infection.

The past medical history is non – contributory. He attends day care with 3 other boys who are all in good health according to the mother.

She is very frustrated because the child has been miserable, complaining of a belly-ache and that his legs hurt. She wants you to "take care of this infection".

*(Continued on next page)*

*(Continued from previous page)*

PHYSICAL EXAM-

T 39.5 HR 180 RR 55

General – The boy appears to be irritable and very uncomfortable
HEENT – TM non-injected with good mobility, conjunctiva are injected with no exudate
Throat – mild erythema but difficult to examine, oral mucosa and lips are dry with some cracking of the skin on the lips

Neck – Supple, + palpable anterior cervical lymph nodes which are firm on exam
Card – S1 S2, No murmur
Skin – Positive Rash, which is raised but blanches well

Extremities- non-pitting edema of the hands and feet

*(Continued on next page)*

*(Continued from previous page)*

LABS-

Rapid Strep- negative

Mono Spot-negative

Blood Culture Pending

CBC –

WBC – 15.6

60 % Neutrophils, 30% Lymphocytes

Platelet Count – 420

H/H – 32/11.5

Erythrocyte sedimentation rate- 55 mm/h

LFT

ALT level is 100 U/L

AST, 295 U/L

Alkaline phosphatase, 171 U/L

Cardiac Echo – unremarkable

## Question 1:

**The most important next step in management would be:**

A) IVIG 2g/Kg
B) High dose acetaminophen for 6-8 weeks
C) IV Corticosteroids
D) IV Ceftriaxone
E) Oral Doxycycline

## Question 2:

**The most likely etiological agent causing the above symptoms would be:**

A) *Rickettsia rickettsii*
B) Epstein-Barr Virus
C) Group A Beta Hemolytic Strep
D) Strep Viridans
E) Unknown

# Case 43

(see page 493 for Answers)

A 3-year-old girl presents with a one-week history of cough and rhinorrhea and a new temperature of 103.9°F. Today she has developed increased respiratory distress along with expiratory stridor that is quite frightening to the parents and her cough is now brassy and productive. A chest x-ray reveals patchy infiltrate and an atypical tracheal air column. The child's immunization status is up to date and she has otherwise been healthy.

## Question 1:

**Which of the following would be the most appropriate immediate next step in managing this patient?**

A) Bronchoscopy to clear secretions and antibiotic coverage for *Staph aureus*
B) Direct laryngoscopy and intubation in the OR
C) Dexamethasone
D) Racemic epinephrine
E) Dexamethasone and racemic epinephrine

## Question 2:

**The most likely diagnosis in this patient would be:**

A) Acute exacerbation of Asthma
B) Acute epiglottitis
C) Viral croup
D) Bacterial tracheitis
E) Foreign body aspiration

# Case 44

*(see page 495 for Answers)*

You are seeing an afebrile 6-year-old boy in the emergency department with a 2-day history of cough and rhinorrhea. His parents report that he is coughing a lot but can't seem to "cough up any mucous" resulting in coughing spasms. In the ER you note that his cough is weak. In the afternoon, he has a difficult time opening his eyes, although this does not seem to be a problem in the morning when he wakes up. On the weekends he is able to walk around and play with other children but he poops out in the early afternoon and hangs out with adults.

His past medical history is unremarkable and his immunizations are up to date.

*(Continued on next page)*

*(Continued from previous page)*

On physical exam he is an alert, responsive boy. He has a difficult time speaking, swallows with difficulty and has diminished gag reflex. EOMI, PERRLA, bilateral ptosis.

His lungs are clear without wheezing, rales or rhonchi. His neurological exam is remarkable for decreased strength in all 4 extremities with normal deep tendon reflexes.

CXR – clear with no infiltrates

CBC – WBC 6.5 with a normal differential

Blood Culture pending

 

## Question 1:

**Which of the following would be most helpful in establishing the correct diagnosis?**

A) MRI of Spine
B) Electromyography
C) Lyme titers
D) Edrophonium test
E) Lumbar puncture

## Question 2:

**Which of the following is the most likely diagnosis?**

A) Transverse myelitis
B) Lyme disease
C) Guillain-Barré Syndrome
D) Myasthenia Gravis
E) Botulism

## Question 3:

**Which of the following will result in marked improvement of the patient's symptoms?**

A) Erythromycin
B) Pyridostigmine
C) Atropine
D) Ceftriaxone
E) Doxycycline

# Case 45

*(see page 499 for Answers)*

You are asked to consult on a 9-month-old boy who presents with respiratory distress.

Past medical history is positive for recurrent otitis media. The baby was born by spontaneous vaginal delivery, which was uneventful. The mother's prenatal care is unknown.

PHYSICAL EXAM:

Afebrile, RR 55, Oxygen Saturations 88-91% on room air.

Weight – Below the 5th percentile for age.

HEENT- EOMI, PERRLA, Ears with scarring on TMs bilaterally. Throat clear

*(Continued on next page)*

*(Continued from previous page)*

Neck – Supple, positive cervical adenopathy

Lungs – Clear

Abdomen- Liver palpable 4 cm below the costal margin with a palpable spleen

CXR- Hyperinflation and bilateral perihilar infiltrates with no consolidation noted.

 

## Question 1:

**Which of the following would suggest a diagnosis of HIV?**

A) Hypergammaglobulinemia
B) Thrombocytosis
C) Leukocytosis
D) Elevated CD4/CD8 ratio
E) Low alanine aminotransferase level

## Question 2:

**You suspect that the x-ray findings may be due to *Pneumocystis carinii* (PCP). Which of the following are true regarding PCP?**

A) Successful treatment with ceftriaxone rules out the diagnosis
B) Serial CXR helps confirm the diagnosis
C) The child should be started immediately on trimethoprim-sulfamethoxazole prophylaxis
D) Confirmation by polymerase chain reaction confirms the diagnosis of *Pneumocystis carinii*
E) The diagnosis of *Pneumocystis carinii* is confirmed by bronchioalveolar lavage (BAL)

 

# Case 46

*(see page 503 for Answers)*

You are asked to evaluate a 4-year-old boy who was diagnosed with ADHD last year. He was started on methylphenidate 5 mg a day, which has not improved his behavior. His parents claim that he is a "very anxious child". You notice that he speaks in a high pitched tone, repeats a lot of the same phrases and is very playful. His attention span is short even when factoring in his age.

On physical exam you note that his head circumference is > 95th%ile with thickened nasal bridge, protruding ears and an elongated face and pointed chin, simian creases are noted on both hands and his testicles are unusually large with an SMR of 1.

## Question 1:

**These findings are most consistent with a diagnosis of:**

A) Autism
B) ADHD
C) Fragile X syndrome
D) William syndrome
E) Precocious puberty

## Question 2:

**Which of the following would confirm the suspected diagnosis?**

A) Karyotype
B) Molecular genetic analysis
C) Serum uric acid levels
D) Referral to a Pervasive developmental center
E) Trial of atomoxetine

## Question 3:

**Long-term management of this patient would consist of:**

A) Behavioral modification and methylphenidate
B) Behavioral modification and atomoxetine
C) Risperdal
D) Multidisciplinary management and care
E) Enzyme replacement therapy

# Case 47

(see page 505 for Answers)

A Caucasian 6-week-old boy is brought in because of severe dehydration that has gotten progressively worse over the past 3 days.
He weighs approximately one pound less than his birth weight and has developed non-bloody diarrhea.
The diarrhea has no mucous and is normal in appearance and texture.
The infant has remained afebrile with no vomiting although at 10 days of life he was switched to a soy based formula because of loose stools and 2 episodes of vomiting.

There is no family history of any metabolic disorders. He is currently on soy formula. The birth history is unremarkable.

*(Continued on next page)*

*(Continued from previous page)*

On physical exam the baby is lethargic, somewhat hypotonic and cyanotic with a shrill cry that makes the entire department's hair stand on end. He appears to be cachectic. He is afebrile with a HR of 180, respiratory rate of 65, and BP of 86/35. His weight is below the 5%ile for age. His pulse oximetry is 85% and does not improve with supplemental oxygen.

HEENT- dry mucous membranes, flat anterior fontanelle with sunken eyes and poor tear production while crying

Lungs- Clear with nasal flaring and mild respiratory distress
Card – S1 S2 no murmur, weak peripheral pulses with a cap refill of 3-4 seconds

*(Continued on next page)*

 

*(Continued from previous page)*

Abdomen- soft, non-tender, no hepatomegaly
GU- normal male genitalia with both testes descended

LABS-

CBC- WBC – 19.5, 20% Neutrophils 10% bands 40% lymphocytes
Lytes, Na/ 129, K/5.0 Cl/109 Bicarb/15
Bun/ 30 Cre/0.4 Glucose/ 110
Blood Culture sent

Lumbar puncture-no evidence of spinal meningitis
RSV- negative

CXR- no consolidation or cardiomegaly
ABG- although the sample was drawn from the radial artery the blood appeared to be venous, even brown in color
pH 7.21/ CO2 18/ O2/ 200

 

## Question 1:

**Which of the following is the most appropriate next step in treating this patient?**

A) Cardiac Echo
B) Intubation
C) IV antibiotics and normal saline bolus
D) Head CT
E) Obtain serum 17-hydroxyprogesterone level

## Question 2:

**Which of the following is the most likely explanation for the child's condition?**

A) Congenital heart disease
B) Bronchiolitis
C) Carbon monoxide exposure
D) Congenital adrenal hyperplasia
E) Methemoglobinemia

## Question 3:

**Which of the following is the most likely explanation for the child's condition?**

A) Prostaglandin drip
B) Aerosolized racemic epinephrine
C) Methylene blue
D) Hyperbaric oxygenation
E) IV hydrocortisone and hydration

# Case 48

(see page 509 for Answers)

You are evaluating a new patient to your practice that is 4 months old. He was born in Honduras and just arrived in the U.S. last month. His birth history is unknown and his medical records are unknown. On physical exam you note that the sutures are widely separated and the patient has a protruding tongue and coarse facial features. The rest of the physical exam is unremarkable except for an umbilical hernia, which is easily reducible.

## Question 1:

**Which of the following would be the most appropriate study?**

A) Karyotype
B) Thyroid function
C) Urine mucopolysaccharoid level
D) Slit lamp eye exam
E) Head CT

## Question 2:

**The most likely diagnosis in his patient would be:**

A) Craniosynostosis
B) Morquio syndrome
C) Hunter Syndrome
D) Hurler Syndrome
E) Hypothyroidism

# Case 49

(see page 511 for Answers)

You are evaluating a 5-month-old infant with fine hair and a crusted rash that is concentrated around the face, hands and feet over the past 3 weeks. The infant has also not gained any weight over the past month and has been less energetic than usual and his stools have been loose, occasionally watery. He has been exclusively breast fed until 4 weeks ago when he was switched to iron based formula in anticipation of the mother returning to work.

## Question 1:

**What is the most likely diagnosis to explain this presentation?**

A) Cow milk allergy
B) Impetigo
C) Cystic fibrosis
D) Celiac Sprue
E) Acrodermatitis enteropathica

## Question 2:

**Which of the following therapeutic interventions are most likely to result in clinical improvement?**

A) Mupirocin cream
B) Pancreatic enzyme replacement
C) Elemental Formula
D) Gluten free diet
E) Zinc supplements

## Question 3:

**The infant is also at risk for which of the following?**

A) Hypogammaglobulinemia
B) Respiratory compromise
C) Asthma
D) Phrynoderma
E) Follicular hyperkeratosis

# Case 50

*(see page 513 for Answers)*

You are asked to consult on a 7-year-old girl because of development of fine pubic hair and hair on the inner thigh with breast budding.
Until recently she has been at the 50th percentile for weight and height but over the past 6 months has experienced an increase in height velocity.
She is taking no medications and has not been exposed to any drugs or toxins. She has not experienced any recent head trauma.
She does not use any makeup.

## Question 1:

**Which of the following would be the most appropriate initial study in establishing a diagnosis?**

A) CT head
B) Abdominal CT
C) Testosterone level
D) Estrogen level
E) Wrist x-ray

## Question 2:

**Which of the following is the most likely explanation for the physical findings?**

A) Exogenous estrogen exposure
B) Exogenous testosterone exposure
C) Idiopathic early maturation of the hypothalamic pathway
D) Adrenal tumor
E) Pituitary tumor

# Case 51

*(see page 515 for Answers)*

A 14-year-old girl presents with a 2-month history of pale patches on her skin, which is very concerning to her. On physical exam you note that the rash is limited to her chest and back and consists of hypopigmented scaling macules with several of them coalescing into patches with distinct borders. She has no history of atopic dermatitis or any other dermatological disorders.

## Question 1:

**The most likely diagnosis is:**

A) Tinea versicolor
B) Tinea corporis
C) Pityriasis rosea
D) Pityriasis alba
E) Vitiligo

## Question 2:

**This is most likely due to:**

A) *Pityrosporum orbiculare*
B) Post inflammatory hypopigmentation
C) Idiopathic hypopigmentation
D) Allergic dermatitis
E) Bacterial superinfection

## Question 3:

**The most appropriate treatment for this patient would be:**

A) Topical antifungal agent
B) Topical steroid
C) Prednisone
D) Avoiding offending agent
E) Cephalexin

# Case 52

*(see page 517 for Answers)*

You are evaluating a 6-week-old infant with increasing levels of respiratory distress. On physical exam you note high-pitched inspiratory stridor that the parents confirm has been for the most part present since birth. There are no audible murmurs on physical examination and the child has otherwise been doing well.

## Question 1:

**The findings in this infant are *most* consistent with:**

A) Foreign body aspiration
B) Supraglottic mass
C) Intrathoracic mass
D) Vascular compression
E) Subglottic mass

## Question 2:

**The most likely diagnosis in this infant would be:**

A) Laryngomalacia
B) Tracheomalacia
C) Subglottic hemangioma
D) Epiglottitis
E) Laryngeal papillomatosis

 

# Case 53

*(see page 519 for Answers)*

You are asked to evaluate a 15-year-old girl because of significant weight loss over the past 2.5 years when she has dropped from the 40th percentile for weight to the 10th percentile. The weight loss is very concerning to the parents and the girl. She is not taking any medications, has not experienced diarrhea or abdominal pain and has generally been asymptomatic except for occasional low-grade fevers, more than would be typical for her age. She also often feels full and bloated and tends to only have one or sometimes two meals a day. A stool sample is negative for O and P, negative for gross blood, and positive for occult blood.

 

## Question 1:

**Which of the following is the most likely explanation for the weight loss in this patient?**

A) Crohn's Disease
B) Ulcerative colitis
C) Anorexia Nervosa
D) Occult malignancy
E) Depression

## Question 2:

**Which of the following would be an important component in managing this patient?**

A) Colectomy to reduce the risk for malignancy
B) PET scan
C) Antidepressant medication
D) Nutritional rehabilitation
E) Enrollment in an eating disorder program

## Question 3:

**Which of the following complications would be most concerning in this patient?**

A) Hypokalemia
B) Metastatic disease
C) Lower GI hemorrhaging
D) Lower than expected adult height
E) Suicide

# Case 54

*(see page 521 for Answers)*

At the 2-week checkup you note that the infant has bilateral mucopurulent eye discharge with some swelling and erythema of the eyelids. You review the hospital record and note the baby was born by spontaneous vaginal delivery with apgars of 8 and 9 with a normal postnatal course. The baby was full term with a birth weight of 3200 grams. Silver nitrate drops were placed in both eyes. The baby has been otherwise feeding well and has regained birthweight.

 

## Question 1:

**The most likely explanation for the bilateral eye discharge would be:**

A) Inadequate technique when the silver nitrate drops were placed
B) Chemical conjunctivitis
C) Herpes keratitis
D) Dacryostenosis
E) Chlamydia conjunctivitis

## Question 2:

**The most appropriate management for this patient would be:**

A) Intramuscular ceftriaxone
B) Erythromycin ophthalmological ointment
C) Erythromycin ethylsuccinate orally
D) Warm compresses
E) IV acyclovir

## Question 3:

**Which of the following complications is most likely in this patient if left untreated?**

A) Permanent blindness
B) Need for corneal transplant
C) Pneumonia
D) Disseminated herpes
E) Will resolve with palliative management

# Case 55

*(see page 523 for Answers)*

You are called to evaluate a rash on a 3-day-old infant by a frantic mother. On physical exam the child is afebrile, alert, and feeding well in the mother's arms. You note a rash on the face and chest which are erythematous macules measuring around 3 cm with a papule in the center.

The mother's prenatal history was unremarkable and the baby was born full term by normal spontaneous vaginal delivery. The mother does have a past history of genital herpes that has not been active in years.

## Question 1:

**The most likely diagnosis is:**

A) Localized Herpes Simplex
B) Neonatal Acne
C) Staph infection
D) Transient neonatal pustular melanosis
E) Erythema toxicum

## Question 2:

**Which of the following would best help establish the diagnosis?**

A) Tzanck Stain
B) Gram Stain
C) Wright Stain
D) Viral Culture
E) Routine culture

## Question 3:

**The most effective treatment would be:**

A) IV antibiotics
B) IV acyclovir
C) Topical antibiotics
D) Topical acyclovir
E) Reassurance

# Case 56

*(see page 525 for Answers)*

You are taking care of an 18-month-old toddler who attends a day care center four days a week and presents with a several week history of watery diarrhea and moderate weight loss. On physical examination you note abdominal distension and low energy. Prior to this point weight gain has been in the 75th percentile with normal growth and development.

 

## Question 1:

**Which of the following steps would be most appropriate in establishing a diagnosis in this patient?**

A) Small bowel biopsy
B) Serum anti- gliadin level
C) Serum anti Giardia antibody
D) String test for Giardia
E) ELISA stool assay for Giardia

## Question 2:

**The most sensitive test in establishing a diagnosis would be:**

A) Small bowel biopsy
B) Serum anti- gliadin level
C) Serum anti Giardia antibody
D) String test for Giardia
E) ELISA stool assay for Giardia

## Question 3:

**The most appropriate treatment for this patient will most likely be:**

A) No treatment
B) Gluten free diet
C) Amoxicillin clavulanic acid
D) Trimethoprim sulfamethoxazole
E) Metronidazole

# Case 57

*(see page 527 for Answers)*

An 11-year-old boy presents with acute onset of swelling just in front of the ear at the jaw line. A school physical 3 months ago was within normal limits with no evidence of facial swelling or adenopathy.
The patient's immunization status is completely up to date.
Two weeks ago the patient did have a severe gastroenteritis and he was seen in the ER but the parents preferred oral rehydration rather than IV hydration as recommended by the pediatric ER attending.

On physical examination you note marked right sided pre-auricular swelling with tender adenopathy and erythema of the overlying skin.

*(Continued on next page)*

*(Continued from previous page)*

Examination of the oral cavity[1] reveals a swollen red area on the lateral aspect of the floor below the tongue with malodorous discharge.
There is no evidence of dental caries.
Tapping on the lower teeth does not result in any pain or discomfort.

[1] Also known as the mouth.

 

## Question 1:

**The most appropriate next step in this patient would be:**

A) Refer to oral surgeon
B) Refer to pediatric dentist
C) Ultrasound
D) Excisional biopsy
E) Treatment based on presentation

## Question 2:

**The most likely diagnosis in this patient would be:**

A) Mumps
B) Mucoepidermoid carcinoma
C) Bacterial Parotitis
D) Epstein Barr Parotitis
E) Talking Tropical parotitis

## Question 3:

**The most appropriate treatment would be:**

A) Workup for immunodeficiency
B) Oral Cefixime
C) IV Cefixime
D) Oral Amoxicillin/Clavulanate
E) Oral Cefazolin and Sour Lemon Candies

 

# Case 58

(see page 531 for Answers)

You are treating a 5-year-old boy for constipation and intermittent abdominal pain, which has gotten worse over the past 3 months. Over the past weeks he has also been vomiting and not feeling well. The pain is intermittent with no set pattern. The parents can feel the stools and gas in the left lower abdomen just as you have on prior visits. You have given the parents instructions on increasing fiber in the diet, which has helped soften the stool, and decreased the severity of the constipation. You have also had to prescribe a stool softener. However the symptoms soon return as soon as the patient is taken off of stool softeners.

The boy has otherwise done fairly well

*(Continued on next page)*

*(Continued from previous page)*

with no significant weight loss or fever. He is taking no medications at this time.

PHYSICAL EXAMINATION

Afebrile, HR 110, RR – 16

Blood pressure 119/ 82

HEENT – PERRLA, TMs intact, and throat clear
Neck – Supple, no palpable lymph nodes

Lungs- Clear, no rhonchi, wheeze or rales

Abdomen – Positive normal bowel sounds, Left lower quadrant pain with radiation to the left flank.
In the left lower abdomen you palpate a firm non-tender mass. No guarding or rebound tenderness.

*(Continued on next page)*

*(Continued from previous page)*

Rectal exam – negative

LAB RESULTS

CBC –

WBC- 9.5 with a normal differential
H/H 12/34

Urinalysis

RBC- 7-10
WBC- 2
Negative Bacteria

Abdominal x-ray – Non-obstructive pattern, hazy left sided mass that appears to be impacted stools

## Question 1:

**The most appropriate imaging procedure on this patient would be:**

A) Abdominal CT Scan with PO contrast
B) Abdominal CT Scan with PO and IV contrast
C) Ultrasound Gallbladder
D) Renal ultrasound
E) Air Contrast enema

## Question 2:

**Once your suspicions are confirmed with the above initial study, the most appropriate followup study would be:**

A) Abdominal CT scan with PO contrast
B) Abdominal CT scan with IV contrast
C) Renal ultrasound
D) Rectal biopsy
E) No study if the initial study is both diagnostic and therapeutic

## Question 3:

**Which of the following additional findings are most likely in this patient?**

A) Aniridia
B) Currant Jelly stools
C) Hypercalcuria
D) Hyperuricemia
E) Aganglionic cells on rectal biopsy

# Case 59

*(see page 535 for Answers)*

You are evaluating an 8 year old boy who according to the parents has been experiencing inappropriate flatulence and abdominal pain on weekend when he is out with friend in the park, particularly during the summer. He is very popular with a group that plays little league baseball and other than an ice cream party after his 2 games on Saturday and Sunday his diet is good. He has been diagnosed with atopic dermatitis which is kept under control with emollient cremes and he has not experienced any flare-ups in several years.

He drinks small amounts of milk occasionally and some dairy products with no difficulty although he tends to shy away from this.

 

## Question 1:

**The most likely explanation for the symptoms is**

A) Behavioral
B) Carbonated beverages
C) Enzyme deficiency
D) IgE mediated allergy
E) IgG mediated allergy

## Question 2:

**The most appropriate treatment would be:**

A) Allergy testing
B) Eliminate dairy products
C) Cut back on carbonated beverages
D) Slowly introduce dairy products
E) Lactase supplements

 

# Case 60

(see page 537 for Answers)

A 15-year-old girl has been experiencing recurrent headaches with increasing frequency.
The headaches are bilateral and feel like a non-pulsating vise-grips tightening on both sides of her head. There has not been any recent head injury. She has not experienced any photophobia or nausea and she is able to carry out routine activities despite the pain.

Her school performance has not changed despite it being difficult to concentrate because of the pain.
She is very concerned about final exams coming up and has had a difficult time managing time.

*(Continued on next page)*

*(Continued from previous page)*

On physical examination the patient appears to be a bit anxious about her final exams. There is no papilledema; cranial nerves are within normal limits. Muscle tone and gait are within normal limits with 2+ deep tendon reflexes throughout.

## Question 1:

**The most appropriate next step for this patient would be:**

A) Referral for psychological counseling
B) Referral for psychiatric treatment
C) Head CT
D) Head MRA
E) Referral for ophthalmological evaluation

## Question 2:

**Which of the following diagnoses would best explain the patient's presentation?**

A) Tension headaches
B) Benign exertional headache
C) Migraine headaches
D) Pseudotumor cerebri
E) Subdural hematoma

## Question 3:

**The most appropriate treatment for this patient would be**

A) Analgesics and relaxation exercises
B) Reduce physical activity
C) Sumatriptan (Imitrex®)
D) Referral to Pediatric Oncologist
E) Corrective lenses

 

# Case 61

(see page 541 for Answers)

You are evaluating an afebrile 13-month-old with a pruritic rash that started 2 weeks earlier and has been getting progressively worse.
Although he has been fussy he has otherwise been asymptomatic.
He was started on whole milk a week before his first birthday.
He has never had any rash before.
He lives with his mother, father, 5-year-old brother and 3-year-old sister; they have no rash or other concerning symptoms.

On physical exam the rash is present on his trunk and extremities including the palms and soles of his feet.
On the trunk you note even distributed red papules along with pustules on the soles of his feet.

## Question 1:

**The most likely explanation of this rash would be:**

A) Bullous impetigo
B) Herpes Simplex Virus
C) Scabies infestation
D) Milk protein allergy
E) Atopic dermatitis

## Question 2:

**The most appropriate intervention would be:**

A) Permethrin 5 % for the patient
B) Permethrin 5 % for the patient and all family members
C) Acyclovir PO
D) Elimination of while milk
E) Amoxicillin Clavulanic acid

## Question 3:

**Two weeks after treatment the rash is reduced in severity and scope and no new lesions appear but the patient is still pruritic (and irritable as a result). The most appropriate treatment at this point would be:**

A) Permethrin 5% for the patient and all household contacts
B) Diphenhydramine
C) Allergy testing
D) Steam clean and hermetically seal all bedding and pets
E) Cephalexin

# Case 62

(see page 543 for Answers)

A 6-year-old boy is brought to your office by his frantic parents because they believe he is having a stroke. They returned 2 days earlier from a camping trip and the boy has otherwise been doing fine. He experienced no recent head trauma and his growth and development have been normal. The parents note that he has never even had a headache before.

On physical examination the boy seems to be hypersensitive to sound and his right eyelid is opened. He is unable to keep it closed when you ask him to resist your attempts to open it. He has no trouble opening both eyes and his extraocular eye movements are intact. When you ask him to smile he

*(Continued on next page)*

 

*(Continued from previous page)*

can only smile on the left side.

His hearing and vision are completely normal.

He can't taste food on the anterior portion of his tongue and there is pain just below his right ear. The patient is experiencing no vertigo or dizziness.

 

## Question 1:

**The most likely diagnosis in this patient would be:**

A) Guillain Barré Syndrome
B) Cerebrovascular accident
C) CNS tumor
D) Migraine headache
E) Neuroborreliosis

## Question 2:

**Which of the following studies will most likely identify the cause of the symptoms?**

A) Head CT
B) Head MRI
C) Lumbar puncture
D) EMG
E) Lyme titers

## Question 3:

**The expected prognosis for this patient would be:**

A) Dependent on staging of tumor
B) Poor if the cerebrovascular accident is hemorrhagic
C) Good if the cerebrovascular accident is vascular
D) Excellent if respiratory support is implemented
E) Excellent with full recovery within a few weeks

# Case 63

*(see page 547 for Answers)*

An 8-year-old boy presents with a patchy distribution of hair loss over the past 8 weeks. On physical exam you note several area of hair loss with the exposed skin exhibiting a scaling appearance with black dots interspersed in some. The rest of the physical exam is unremarkable.

 

## Question 1:

**The most likely diagnosis is:**

A) Alopecia neurotica
B) Trichotillomania
C) Alopecia areata
D) Tinea capitis
E) Tension alopecia

## Question 2:

**This can be best diagnosed by:**

A) Wright Stain
B) Wrong Stain
C) Gram Stain
D) Tzanck Stain
E) Potassium Hydroxide Preparation

## Question 3:

**The most appropriate treatment would be:**

A) Topical antibiotics
B) Oral antibiotics
C) Topical antifungal cream
D) Oral Antifungal
E) Stress reduction measures

# Case 64

(see page 549 for Answers)

A 12-year-old boy has been gradually experiencing difficulty walking. On physical exam you note a hammer toe in the right foot with some atrophy of the muscles over the dorsal aspect of both feet as well as high arches bilaterally. The muscles of the legs appear to have moderate tone with what can best be described as a stork-like appearance. The muscles of the hands appear to be atrophied as well and look like "claw hands".
Deep tendon reflexes are diminished in all 4 extremities. There is a negative Babinski sign.

His growth and development have otherwise been normal. There is a family history for a muscle weakness but the parents are not clear on the details.

 

## Question 1:

**Which of the following would be most useful in *initially* establishing the correct diagnosis?**

A) EMG
B) Tensilon study
C) Muscle Biopsy
D) Genetic karyotyping
E) Serum creatinine kinase level

## Question 2:

**Which of the following diagnoses is the most likely explanation for the patient's presentation?**

A) Guillain Barré Disease
B) Charcot-Marie –Tooth Disease
C) Friedreich Ataxia
D) Becker's muscular dystrophy
E) Duchenne's muscular dystrophy

# Case 65

(see page 551 for Answers)

You are taking care of a 5-year-old boy in the 10th %ile for height. In addition you note bowing of the legs.
His balanced diet has been documented by a nutritionist.

Laboratory findings include
normal parathyroid hormone level.
Serum calcium is 9.7, phosphorus 3.0, alkaline phosphatase of 790.
Vitamin D 25 hydroxy is normal;
Vitamin D 1, 25 dihydroxy is low.

 

## Question 1:

**The most likely etiology for this patient's presentation would be:**

A) Hypoparathyroidism
B) Nutritional rickets
C) Vitamin D dependent rickets
D) Vitamin D deficiency rickets
E) Familial hypophosphatemic rickets

## Question 2:

**The most effective treatment would be :**

A) Calcitriol supplementation
B) Cholecalciferol supplementation
C) Calcium supplementation
D) Phosphorus supplementation
E) Parathyroidectomy

# Case 66

(see page 555 for Answers)

You are called to evaluate a rash on a 3-day-old infant by a frantic mother. On physical exam the child is afebrile, alert, and feeding well in the mother's arms. You note a rash on the face and chest which is pustular with an erythematous base along with several hyperpigmented macules which include a collarette of scale.

The mother's prenatal history was unremarkable and the baby was born full term by normal spontaneous vaginal delivery. The mother does have a past history of genital herpes, which has not been active in years.

## Question 1:

**The most likely diagnosis is:**

A) Localized Herpes Simplex
B) Neonatal Acne
C) Staph infection
D) Transient neonatal pustular melanosis
E) Erythema toxicum

## Question 2:

**Which of the following would best help establish the diagnosis?**

A) Tzanck Stain
B) Gram Stain
C) Potassium hydroxide preparation
D) Viral Culture
E) Routine culture

## Question 3:

**The most effective treatment would be:**

A) IV antibiotics
B) IV acyclovir
C) Topical antibiotics
D) Topical acyclovir
E) Reassurance

 

# Case 67

(see page 557 for Answers)

An 8-year-old boy presents with a patchy distribution of hair loss over the past 8 weeks. On physical exam you note one area of hair loss with hair of varying length.
There are no broken hairs noted and no erythema, scaling or black dots noted.
The rest of the physical exam is unremarkable.

 

## Question 1:

**The most likely diagnosis is :**

A) Alopecia neurotica
B) Trichotillomania
C) Alopecia areata
D) Tinea capitis
E) Tension alopecia

## Question 2:

**The most appropriate treatment would be:**

A) Topical antibiotics
B) Oral antibiotics
C) Topical antifungal cream
D) Oral Antifungal
E) Stress reduction measures

 

# Case 68

(see page 559 for Answers)

A 16-year-old ingested a "fistful of pills" according to the group that brought her to the emergency room. She was non-responsive in the field and was intubated as a precaution. Your initial lab results include a toxicology screen positive for benzodiazepines and for acetaminophen. Liver function studies are pending. She was witnessed ingesting the pills 2 hours ago.

## Question 1:

**Which of the following can be seen during the first 24 hours following a toxic ingestion of acetaminophen?**

A) Asymptomatic
B) Encephalopathy
C) Hyperbilirubinemia
D) Bleeding abnormalities
E) Elevated LFT's

## Question 2:

**Which of the following would be true regarding the initial management of this patient?**

A) Administration of N-Acetylcysteine should be started
B) Administration of N-Acetylcysteine should be delayed based on the results of the Liver function studies
C) Administration of N-Acetylcysteine should be delayed based on an acetaminophen level in 2 hours.
D) Administration of N-Acetylcysteine should be delayed based on a repeat acetaminophen level in 4 hours

 

## Question 3:

**Additional management of this patient could include:**

A) Avoiding activated charcoal since it will interfere with absorption of N-Acetylcysteine
B) Administer Flumazenil immediately
C) Administer Flumazenil only after LFT results are back
D) Administer Flumazenil only after repeat acetaminophen level is back
E) Flumazenil would be contraindicated in this scenario

 

# Case 69

(see page 561 for Answers)

You are evaluating a 4-year-old boy with a history of atopic dermatitis who presents with a severe rash on the extensor surface of his legs with a milder appearing rash on his arms and trunk. The rash can be best described as thin scales that have a pasted-on appearance with an elevated edge.

The boy's father has a very similar appearing rash and there is a strong family history of asthma and allergies to environmental agents.

 

## Question 1:

**The most likely explanation for this child's rash is:**

A) Secondarily infected atopic dermatitis
B) Food allergy
C) Poorly controlled atopic dermatitis
D) Contact dermatitis
E) Ichthyosis vulgaris

## Question 2:

**The best initial treatment of this rash would be:**

A) Cephalexin
B) Elimination of offending agent
C) Triamcinolone 0.1%
D) Prednisone
E) Emollients

## Question 3:

**This condition is inherited in which pattern?**

A) Autosomal recessive
B) Autosomal dominant
C) X- Linked recessive
D) X- Linked dominant
E) Random

# Case 70

*(see page 563 for Answers)*

A 3-year-old was found spitting out the contents of an opened bottle containing a liquid outdoor cleaner which is known to contain an acidic caustic substance. On physical examination the child is in no distress and you note that there are no lesions on the oral mucosa or pharynx.

## Question 1:

**Which of the following would be the most appropriate intervention?**

A) Oral hydration
B) IV hydration
C) Nasogastric lavage
D) Activated charcoal
E) Activated charcoal with sorbitol

## Question 2:

**Which of the following is true regarding the ingestion of caustic substances?**

A) The extent of tissue damage is directly related to the volume ingested
B) Alkali ingestion is associated with a higher risk for perforation
C) Acid ingestions is associated with a higher risk for perforation
D) The absence of oropharyngeal lesions lowers the risk for esophageal injury
E) The absence of drooling, dysphagia and chest pain rules out esophageal injury

## Question 3:

**Over the next two days which of the following should be done regardless of clinical progress**

A) IV hydration
B) Oral rehydration
C) Endoscopy
D) Colonoscopy
E) All steps should be based on clinical progress

# Case 71

(see page 565 for Answers)

You are doing a school physical on a 15-year-old boy. He consistently gets A's and B's. His cardiac exam is normal although he does have a pectus excavatum, which the mother confided in you earlier that he is self-conscious about. He has previously participated and even excelled in sports but upon entering high school has withdrawn from all sports activity and is frequently out of breath while engaging in any activity at home or with close friends.

## Question 1:

**The most likely explanation for the boy's reluctance to participate in sports and dyspnea would be:**

A) Poor pulmonary function secondary to pectus excavatum
B) Exercise induced asthma
C) Aortic dilatation
D) Clinical depression
E) Lack of exercise

## Question 2:

**The most appropriate management of this patient would be**

A) Albuterol via MDI prior to engaging in sports activity
B) Guacamole dip for the chest concavity to help his transition from participant to spectator
C) Psychotherapy and antidepressants
D) Cardiac Echo
E) Reassurance and encouragement to participate in sports

# Case 72

*(see page 567 for Answers)*

You are called to the delivery room to evaluate a ten pound three ounce baby boy delivered vaginally. The delivery, as you could imagine, was difficult with marked shoulder dystocia.

The nurses are concerned because the infant is not moving his right arm well. You note that the baby is maintaining his upper arm in an internally rotated position with the shoulder adducted close to the body with his lower arm pronated and wrist flexed.

## Question 1:

**The most likely diagnosis in this patient is :**

A) Fractured clavicle
B) Erb Palsy
C) Klumpke's Palsy
D) Dislocated shoulder
E) Fractured humerus

## Question 2:

**Another common finding in this patient would be:**

A) Anhidrosis on the right side
B) Anhidrosis of the left side
C) Osteomyelitis
D) Aseptic necrosis of the humeral head
E) Tension pneumothorax

## Question 3:

**The prognosis for this patient would be:**

A) Full recovery within one month
B) Some improvement within one month
C) Spontaneous recovery within a day
D) Permanent deficit in the upper arm
E) Permanent deficit in the lower arm

# Case 73

(see page 569 for Answers)

A 15-year-old boy is brought to your office. He appears to be healthy and is active in several sports. He is alarmed because he woke up in the morning and noticed that his eyes were yellow. However when he returns from school in the afternoon his eyes are white again. However this has been going on for over a week and he is concerned.

He does not drink any alcohol or take drugs, he is not sexually active and has no body piercing or tattoos.
His physical exam is unremarkable including a soft abdomen with no guarding, rebound or hepatosplenomegaly. His bilirubin is 2.3 over 0.1 and his liver function tests are negative. All of his immunizations are up to date including the hepatitis B series which he received at birth.

 

## Question 1:

**The most likely explanation for his presentation would be**

A) Hepatitis A
B) Hepatitis B
C) Hepatitis C
D) Gilbert syndrome
E) Infectious mononucleosis

## Question 2:

**Which of the following would be the most appropriate study to confirm the diagnosis?**

A) Serum hepatitis A antibody
B) Serum hepatitis B surface antigen
C) Followup liver function studies
D) Ebstein Barr titers
E) No further evaluation is necessary

## Question 3:

**The long-term prognosis for this patient is:**

A) 80% chance of developing chronic hepatitis
B) 50% chance of developing chronic hepatitis
C) 75% chance of developing chronic hepatitis
D) Several months to recover followed by full recovery
E) Occasional episodes of mild jaundice otherwise excellent

 

# Case 74

*(see page 571 for Answers)*

An 8-year-old boy is new to your practice. The mother heard about your stellar reputation and excellent taste in starchy white coats and tacky novelty ties. Her concern is over her son's repeated sinus infections with no explanations provided by the previous pediatrician whose lack of taste in ties rivals and usually exceeds yours. His old chart arrives on your desk with a thud that knocks your CD collection off the hanging plastic CD holder.

You note that in the past 3 years he has had 6 sinus infections and a few ear infections. Height and weight are in the 75th percentile for age and his development is within normal limits.

## Question 1:

**The most likely explanation for this patient's history would be:**

A) T Cell mediated immunodeficiency
B) HIV
C) Agammaglobulinemia
D) Nasal polyps
E) Chronic allergic rhinitis

## Question 2:

**The most appropriate management for this patient would be:**

A) Chronic low dose antibiotics
B) HIV testing and counseling
C) Measurement of serum immunoglobulins
D) Sweat testing
E) Trial of intranasal steroids

# Case 75

*(see page 573 for Answers)*

You are evaluating a 13-year-old boy for severe chest pain and shortness of breath. He is enrolled in a special education program because according to the parents "he is slow".

On physical examination he is thin for his age with scoliosis.

Ophthalmological examination reveals posterior displaced lenses.

There is a normal S1 S2 with no murmurs or gallops noted. Capillary refill is less than 2 seconds.

He is afebrile with a pulse of 92 and respiratory rate of 64. Portable chest x-ray is negative.

## Question 1:

**The most appropriate next step in this patient would be:**

A) Cardiac Stress test
B) Standard chest x-ray when the patient is stabilized
C) Intubation
D) Chest x-ray
E) Chest CT

## Question 2:

**The most immediate cause of the patient's symptoms is:**

A) Pulmonary embolus
B) Cardiomyopathy
C) Pericarditis
D) Pericardial effusion
E) Pleurisy

## Question 3:

**Which of the following diagnoses best explains the patient's overall findings?**

A) Marfan Syndrome
B) Klinefelter's syndrome
C) Noonan syndrome
D) Homocystinuria
E) Hurler Syndrome

# Case 76

(see page 575 for Answers)

At the 2-week followup visit you notice that the neonate is slightly icteric. You review the neonatal record and discover that he had mild physiological jaundice which resolved after 5 days. He has already surpassed his birth weight, is breast-feeding well and producing loose mustard colored stools on a regular basis.

On physical examination he is icteric down to the thighs with symmetrical muscle tone and strength and is alert and responsive. Abdomen is soft, non-tender with no hepatosplenomegaly.

His total and direct bilirubin is 18/ 0.5

 

## Question 1:

**The most likely cause of the baby's color is:**

A) Excessive beta carotene ingestion
B) Galactosemia
C) Congenital CMV
D) Breast milk jaundice
E) Jaundice associated with breastfeeding

## Question 2:

**The most appropriate management of this baby's condition would be:**

A) Phototherapy
B) Galactose free diet
C) Discontinue breastfeeding indefinitely
D) Discontinue breastfeeding for 48 hours then resume
E) Ultrasound of liver

## Question 3:

**The percentage of infants who experience jaundice for the same condition is closest to:**

A) 90% or more
B) 75% or more
C) 25% or more
D) 10% or more
E) Less than 2%

# Case 77

(see page 577 for Answers)

A 3-year-old toddler was found with an opened bottle of over–the-counter 200 mg ibuprofen tablets with half chewed tablets in his mouth. The ingestion occurred roughly 4 hours ago.
The child weighs 15 kg and there were twenty pills in the bottle and sixteen are left. On physical examination the child is comfortable eating ice cream and remains playful. Vital signs are stable.

 

## Question 1:

**What would be the most appropriate management at this point?**

A) Syrup of ipecac
B) Activated charcoal with sorbitol
C) Activated charcoal without sorbitol
D) Nasogastric lavage
E) Observation only

## Question 2:

**Which of the following laboratory studies would be indicated at this time?**

A) Ibuprofen levels at this time and repeat in two hours
B) Ibuprofen levels in two hours
C) Liver function studies
D) CBC and electrolytes
E) Observation only

## Question 3:

**Each of the following is a possible finding in ibuprofen toxicity *except for*:**

A) Diplopia
B) Acute respiratory distress syndrome
C) Apnea
D) Seizures
E) Nausea

# Case 78

(see page 579 for Answers)

You are evaluating a 6-year-old girl who is experiencing abdominal pain without any nausea or diarrhea.
In addition she has been experiencing urinary frequency and diurnal enuresis with no dysuria. On physical exam there is left lower quadrant tenderness with no guarding or rebound with increased bowel sounds.

 

## Question 1:

**The most appropriate next study to order in this patient would be:**

A) Plain abdominal film
B) Urinalysis and Urine Culture
C) Renal ultrasound
D) Abdominal CT with IV contrast
E) Abdominal CT with oral contrast

## Question 2:

**The most likely diagnosis is:**

A) Neurogenic bladder
B) Encopresis
C) Urinary tract infection
D) Vesicoureteral reflux
E) Diabetes Melitis

## Question 3:

**The most appropriate management for this patient would be:**

A) Spinal MRI
B) Increased dietary fiber
C) Trimethoprim sulfamethoxazole
D) VCUG study
E) Measure serum glucose

# Case 79

(see page 581 for Answers)

An 8-year-old boy presents with severe right-sided ear pain of one week's duration that has interfered with his sleep. He plays goalie for his ice hockey team on a regular basis and wears protective equipment and does not recall sustaining any significant trauma. The pain radiates to the chin and neck and improves somewhat with ibuprofen but never fully.

He has had no sore throat symptoms, nasal discharge, dysphagia, or discharge from the ear. On physical examination there is no tenderness on movement of the outer ear, there is a clear view of the tympanic membrane with no inflammation and a positive light reflex with all landmarks visible. The throat is clear with no erythema or exudate noted. No oral lesions noted.

## Question 1:

**The most likely diagnosis to explain the patient's symptoms would be:**

A) Hunt syndrome
B) Otitis Externa
C) Serous Otitis media
D) Temporomandibular joint syndrome
E) Herpes zoster oticus

## Question 2:

**The most appropriate next step in managing this patient would be :**

A) Referral to a pediatric ENT specialist
B) Stop participation in all contact sports immediately
C) Nasal decongestants and oral antibiotics
D) Oral Acyclovir
E) Dental workup

# Case 80

*(see page 583 for Answers)*

You are evaluating a 14-year-old basketball player who twisted his ankle coming down for a rebound. He arrived in your office bearing weight with a significant limp. On physical examination you note pain and swelling over the lateral ankle with both passive and active movement. You do not see any evidence of a fracture on x-ray.

 

## Question 1:

**Which of the following would be the most appropriate next step?**

A) Continue weight bearing as tolerated
B) Light weight bearing as tolerated
C) Splint with no weight bearing
D) Ace bandage and return to full activity as tolerated
E) Ace Bandage and light activity

## Question 2:

**Which of the following would be the greatest concern at this point?**

A) Salter Harris 1 Fracture
B) Salter Harris 2 Fracture
C) Salter Harris 3 Fracture
D) Salter Harris 4 Fracture
E) Severe sprain

## Question 3:

**Each of the following would be appropriate immediate management except for:**

A) Elevation
B) Avoid weight bearing
C) Bandage and splinting
D) Ice
E) Heat

# Case 81

(see page 585 for Answers)

A 6-month-old child presents with a pruritic rash. On physical exam you note scaling of the scalp and the flexural folds of the extremities. There is also a greasy appearance of the scalp lesions. There is no evidence of diaper rash. There is no rash on other family members.

## Question 1:

**The most likely explanation for this rash is:**

A) Atopic dermatitis
B) Scabies infestation
C) Erysipelas
D) Seborrhea
E) Contact dermatitis

## Question 2:

**The most appropriate treatment would be:**

A) Emollients and hydrocortisone 1%
B) Permethrin 5% to patient
C) Permethrin 5% to patient and household contacts
D) Application of baby oil
E) Avoidance of offending agent

 

# Case 82

*(see page 587 for Answers)*

You are evaluating a 15-year-old who is presenting with a sore throat so painful it is difficult to swallow. He has a temperature of 102.4 and you note marked erythema of his pharynx with no exudate and his right tonsil is more swollen than the left, with the uvula shifter to the left. He has no respiratory stridor but is in a great deal of pain.

His immunizations are up to date and he has been otherwise doing well.

## Question 1:

**The most likely diagnosis to explain this patient's presentation would be:**

A) Retropharyngeal abscess
B) Peritonsillar abscess
C) Bacterial tracheitis
D) Epiglottitis
E) Viral croup

## Question 2:

**The most appropriate immediate step in managing this patient would be:**

A) Lateral neck x-ray
B) Endotracheal intubation to protect the airway
C) Incision and drainage
D) Endoscopic suctioning of secretions
E) Racemic epinephrine

## Question 3:

**Once the patient is stabilized the most appropriate management would be:**

A) Continuous racemic epinephrine
B) Oral antibiotic coverage for Staph aureus
C) Oral antibiotic coverage for Group A streptococcus and anaerobes
D) IV antibiotic coverage for Staph aureus
E) IV antibiotic coverage for Group A streptococcus and anaerobes

# Case 83

*(see page 589 for Answers)*

You are evaluating a 2-year-old with "chronic otitis externa" with discharge. Despite a course of ofloxacin otic and appropriate oral antibiotics the otorrhea continues. There is no known history of barotrauma and the parents do not recall anything being placed in the ear. The child is afebrile with normal growth and developmental milestones. On physical examination it is difficult to visualize the tympanic membrane because of cerumen and other debris. There is no pain on manipulation of the outer ear.

## Question 1:

**What is the most likely cause of the persistent otorrhea?**

A) Otitis media
B) Otitis externa
C) Serous otitis
D) Serious Malingering
E) Foreign body

## Question 2:

**The most appropriate management at this point would be:**

A) 2nd course of Ofloxacin
B) Hydrogen peroxide drops followed by 2nd course of Ofloxacin drops
C) Hydrogen peroxide drops followed by 2nd course of oral antibiotics
D) Gentle irrigation of the ear
E) Immediate referral to ENT

# Case 84

(see page 591 for Answers)

You are evaluating a 2-year-old toddler who has been experiencing increasing diarrhea which continues despite several attempts to modify the child's diet. With the exception of the first stool of the day, the stools are loose and malodorous with visible food particles noted during diaper changes. Growth and development are within normal limits for all parameters. His appetite is normal for age.

## Question 1:

**The most likely etiological explanation for the diarrhea is:**

A) Altered gastrointestinal motility
B) Giardia lamblia
C) Lactose intolerance
D) Celiac Sprue
E) Cow milk allergy

## Question 2:

**The most appropriate step in managing this patient would be:**

A) Decrease fat content to below 4 g/kg/day
B) Increase fat content to above 4-6 g/kg/day
C) Increase Carbohydrate content in diet
D) Decrease dairy product intake
E) Serum anti-gliadin level

# Case 85

(see page 593 for Answers)

A 13-month-old child presents with a pruritic rash that has been recurring since the age of 9 months. On physical exam you note large areas of hypopigmentation on the upper extremities, which are scaly and chapped. There is marked scaling on the flexure surfaces. There is no evidence of diaper rash. There is no rash on other family members. Other than asthma the family history is negative.

## Question 1:

**The most likely explanation for this rash is:**

A) Atopic dermatitis
B) Scabies infestation
C) Erysipelas
D) Seborrhea
E) Contact dermatitis

## Question 2:

**The most appropriate treatment would be:**

A) Emollients and hydrocortisone 1%
B) Permethrin 5% to patient
C) Permethrin 5% to patient and household contacts
D) Cephalexin
E) Avoidance of offending agent

 

# Case 86

(see page 595 for Answers)

You are evaluating a full term newborn who is tachypneic with audible rales. He was born via spontaneous vaginal delivery with no complications.

On physical examination pulses to both the arms and legs are diminished and, other than an audible gallop, there are no cardiac murmurs. On cardiac echo systolic ejection fraction is normal and there is no evidence of congenital heart disease. Chest x-ray shows increased vascular markings.

## Question 1:

**Which of the following conditions would best explain the clinical presentation?**

A) Coarctation of the aorta
B) Supracardiac total anomalous pulmonary venous return
C) Intracranial arteriovenous malformation
D) Hepatic arteriovenous malformation
E) Truncus arteriosus communis

## Question 2:

**If left untreated the following outcome would be expected:**

A) Systemic hypertension
B) Diminished left ventricular function
C) Increased left ventricular function
D) Decreased pulmonary blood flow
E) Portal Hypertension

# Case 87

(see page 599 for Answers)

You are caring for a 7-year-old boy who has moved to your area with his family. You review his old chart and notice that he has had 3 episodes of lobar pneumonia requiring hospitalization for several days. In addition he has had one episode of documented osteomyelitis requiring hospitalization. He is afebrile with clear lungs and normal cardiac exam with no murmurs. There are several shoddy submandibular lymph nodes.

His CBC shows a WBC of 12.5 with a normal differential, hematocrit is 32, hemoglobin 11.5 and an MCV of 95. Platelet count is 175K.

 

## Question 1:

**The most likely explanation for this rash is:**

A) Atopic dermatitis
B) Scabies infestation
C) Erysipelas
D) Seborrhea
E) Contact dermatitis

## Question 2:

**The most appropriate treatment would be:**

A) Emollients and hydrocortisone 1%
B) Permethrin 5% to patient
C) Permethrin 5% to patient and household contacts
D) Cephalexin
E) Avoidance of offending agent

# Case 88

*(see page 601 for Answers)*

You are evaluating a 6-year-old boy who has been limping on his left leg for 4 weeks. His history is negative except for a minor fall while playing basketball around the time the limp started.
He has had no recent viral illnesses and there is no significant past medical history.

On physical exam he is afebrile with some pain over the inguinal area increased with abduction of the leg, which is limited.

## Question 1:

**The most appropriate next step in diagnosing the cause of the symptoms?**

A) Serum Lyme titers
B) Tap and culture of the hip
C) Hip CT
D) Serum Rheumatoid factor
E) Frog leg AP x-ray of the pelvis

## Question 2:

**Which of the following is the most likely explanation for the child's condition?**

A) Septic arthritis
B) Toxic synovitis
C) Juvenile rheumatoid arthritis
D) Lyme Disease
E) Legg Calve Perthes disease

# Case 89

(see page 603 for Answers)

You are evaluating a 16-year-old male in the emergency department for chest pain. She describes the pain as being constant and keeping her up at night. Ibuprofen has been of no help–the pain is much worse when he is lying down and he must lie down at an angle in order to sleep. He does much better sitting or standing up and has experienced no shortness of breath. His EKG was normal and his cardiac echo exam showed no compromise in cardiac function.

 

## Question 1:

**The most likely diagnosis to explain this patient's presentation would be:**

A) Myopericarditis
B) Myocarditis
C) Pericarditis
D) Costochondritis
E) Gastroesophageal reflux disease

## Question 2:

**An important complication which may develop would be:**

A) Left bundle branch block
B) Congestive heart failure
C) Pleurisy and empyema
D) Barrett's esophagitis
E) Pericardial tamponade

## Question 3:

**A common etiology of this patient's condition would be:**

A) Adenovirus
B) Borrelia burgdorferi
C) Helicobacter pylori
D) Group A Beta Hemolytic Strep
E) Enterobius vermicularis

 

# Case 90

*(see page 605 for Answers)*

You are evaluating an 18-month-old boy who immigrated from Guatemala two months ago. He presents with a fever of 103.5 F, with a severe cough, inflammation of the nares and rhinorrhea. His eyes are red and inflamed as well. In addition you note a macular rash concentrated behind his ears as well as his face and trunk.

 

## Question 1:

**The symptoms in this patient are most likely due to :**

A) Rubella
B) Rubeola
C) Ruby slippers
D) Parvovirus B19
E) Adenovirus

## Question 2:

**Which of the following supplementations would be indicated in this patient to reduce morbidity and mortality?**

A) Vitamin A
B) Vitamin B 12
C) Vitamin C
D) Vitamin D
E) Vitamin E

# Case 91

(see page 607 for Answers)

You are evaluating a 17-year-old female for a routine physical examination. While taking the history she confirms that she has been sexually active and prefers not to tell her parents. She last had sexual relations 6 weeks ago and once before that with a different partner. She is pretty sure that both boys used condoms. Her last menstrual period was 2 weeks ago. She is not experiencing any dysuria, dysmenorrhea, or abdominal pain. Her urine HCG is negative.

## Question 1:

**Which of the following would be most appropriate for this visit?**

A) Pelvic examination and cultures for Chlamydia, Gonorrhea and serum HCG
B) Pelvic examination and cultures for Chlamydia, Gonorrhea
C) Serum HCG
D) No intervention or counseling regarding sexual activity to maintain privacy
E) Urine DNA amplification test for Gonorrhea and Chlamydia

## Question 2:

**Which of the following is true regarding this patient?**

A) Most low grade squamous intraepithelial lesions in adolescents progress
B) Pap smear is a high priority during health visits for sexually active females
C) American cancer society recommendations include delay of Pap screening until 3 years after onset of sexual activity
D) American cancer society recommendations include delay of Pap screening at the time of onset of sexual activity
E) DNA amplification urine testing has replaced standard PAP smear

 

# Case 92

*(see page 609 for Answers)*

You are evaluating a newborn male. The mother has been breastfeeding the baby every 3 hours as needed. The mother is very concerned because the baby has not passed a stool in 5 days. On physical examination of the baby there are no significant findings and the abdomen is soft and non-tender.

The baby was full-term and delivered by normal spontaneous vaginal delivery with no complications. Apgars were 9 at one minute and five minutes. The baby has lost 4% of his birthweight and he passed a meconium stool within 24 hours.

## Question 1:

**The most appropriate next step would be:**

A) Introduce formula supplementation
B) Abdominal plain film
C) Add Sugar water to the diet
D) Glycerin suppository
E) Reassurance

## Question 2:

**The most likely explanation for the presentation would be:**

A) Insufficient frequency of breast feeding
B) Low initial volume of breast milk
C) Small bowel obstruction
D) Anal atresia
E) Anal stenosis

# Case 93

*(see page 611 for Answers)*

A 16-year-old girl was taking a walk with her sister along the beach during August. Earlier in the day she received a text message from her boyfriend informing her that he was out of state and ending their relationship. While they were walking the girl felt light-headed and quickly sat down and subsequently passed out in her sister's arms. Just before passing out, her face turned red and she was perspiring. The episode lasted less than a minute and you have been asked to evaluate her as a precaution. Except for nausea she has remained asymptomatic since the episode. She was recently started on a tricyclic antidepressant.

Her blood pressure was 119/79 standing and sitting with a pulse rate of 72. She is afebrile. Her EKG showed normal sinus rhythm with no abnormalities noted.

 

## Question 1:

**The most likely explanation for the patient's presentation is:**

A) Conversion reaction
B) Long QT syndrome
C) Heatstroke
D) Heat exhaustion
E) Hyperventilation

## Question 2:

**Which of the following would apply to this patient's situation?**

A) She is at risk for sudden death
B) She needs to be admitted for IV fluid therapy
C) She should remain indoors drinking copious amount of fluids
D) The tricyclic antidepressants should be discontinued immediately
E) Arrangements for inpatient psychiatric care should be made immediately

 

# Case 94

(see page 613 for Answers)

During a routine physical examination a 16-year-old teenager notes that she is very concerned about being overweight.

On physical examination her weight is above the 95th percentile and her heights are in the 92nd percentile for her age. Her neck is supple and there are no palpable masses noted. The rest of her physical examination is unremarkable.

Laboratory studies include a:

CBC 10.5 with a Hematocrit of 39 and hemoglobin 12.5 with normal differential. Her serum sodium is 139, potassium 4.0, Chloride of 107, Bicarb 24, Glucose 90, Bun 25, creatinine 0.8.

*(Continued on next page)*

 

*(Continued from previous page)*

Serum thyroxine level is low but Free T4 levels and TSH are both normal. $T_3$ resin uptake is elevated.

## Question 1:

**The most likely diagnosis in this patient would be:**

A) Anorexia nervosa
B) Hashimoto's thyroiditis
C) Graves disease
D) Thyroid-binding globulin deficiency
E) Primary Hypothyroidism

## Question 2:

**The diagnosis can be best confirmed by:**

A) Psychiatric consultation
B) Serum long acting thyroid stimulating factor
C) Serum antithyroid antibodies
D) Serum thyroid binding globulin levels
E) Needle biopsy

# Case 95

*(see page 617 for Answers)*

You are evaluating a 3-year-old girl in the emergency room who presents with wheezing and respiratory distress with no improvement with 2 albuterol aerosols in the field and one upon arrival in the ED. She is lethargic and diaphoretic with increased salivation. Her eyes are miotic with pupils equal and reactive to light. The wheezing continues but she is able to breath on her own. Her cardiac exam in normal and you note increased bowel sounds. Just prior to this she was playing in her grandfather's garden.

## Question 1:

**The most likely explanation for the presenting symptoms would be:**

A) Foreign body ingestion
B) Organophosphate toxicity
C) Atropine toxicity
D) Ethanol Toxicity
E) Opiate toxicity

## Question 2:

**The most appropriate initial step in managing this patient would be:**

A) Endotracheal intubation
B) Inspiratory /Expiratory Chest X-ray
C) Bronchoscopy
D) IV Atropine
E) Remove clothing and bathe

## Question 3:

**The most appropriate management after stabilization would be:**

A) Subcutaneous epinephrine
B) Racemic epinephrine via nebulizer
C) IM Naloxone
D) IV Atropine
E) IV Lorazepam

# Case 96

(see page 619 for Answers)

You are evaluating a 12-year-old girl who is just getting over an upper respiratory tract infection. The parents note that the cold only lasted 3 days because of the homemade tea she was given. Unfortunately, they arrive in your office frantic as they pull out two specimen cups, one with the patient's urine and the other with the tea and challenge you to distinguish them.

How about that - they look identical! Instead of admitting this you ask for another specimen. The parents note that a similar thing happened 3 months ago, and the other doctor distinguished the two cups by tasting them, fortunately he picked the tea first. You pretend not to hear this as you leave the room for

*(Continued on next page)*

*(Continued from previous page)*

an "emergency". There is no history of fever.

The patient has a low-grade fever. Blood pressure is 110/70 there is no rash, joint pain, edema or any other symptoms.

The WBC is 9.5 with a normal differential. Electrolytes and serum complement levels are normal.

1 Also known as the mouth.

 

## Question 1:

**The most likely diagnosis is:**

A) Hypercalciuria
B) Post strep glomerulonephritis
C) IgA nephropathy
D) Alport syndrome
E) UTI

## Question 2:

**Other possible findings and developments in this patient would include:**

A) Sensironeural hearing loss
B) Vesicoureteral reflux
C) Pulmonary disease
D) Elevated IgA levels
E) Decreased IgA levels

## Question 3:

**The long-term prognosis in this patient is closest to:**

A) 10% chance of end stage renal disease
B) 45% chance of end stage renal disease
C) High risk for development of renal stones
D) Chronic treatment with steroids
E) Short term problem with excellent prognosis

 

# Case 97

*(see page 623 for Answers)*

While playing outdoors with some friends a 7-year-old boy falls down and experiences a witnessed generalized tonic-clonic seizure. By objective accounts the seizure lasts a minute and a half. There was not trauma now nor in the past. Other than a documented febrile seizure at the age of 3 there is no significant neurological history, developmental delay or cognitive impairment.

An EEG done 2 days later demonstrates some left temporal slowing.

## Question 1:

**Which of the following would be most appropriate in the management of this child?**

A) Stat Head CT
B) Stat Head MRI
C) Non-urgent Head MRI
D) Non –urgent Head CT
E) Begin anticonvulsant medications immediately

## Question 2:

**Which of the following is true regarding risk of epilepsy in children experiencing febrile seizures?**

A) There is a 75% greater chance of developing epilepsy than the general population
B) There is a 50% greater chance of developing epilepsy than the general population
C) There is a 25% greater chance of developing epilepsy than the general population
D) There is a 1% greater chance of developing epilepsy than the general population
E) There is no greater chance of developing epilepsy than the general population

## Question 3:

**Which of the following would be indications for implementing anticonvulsant medication?**

A) One prior febrile seizure
B) Two prior febrile seizures
C) One afebrile seizure causing loss of consciousness
D) EEG findings of spike discharges
E) EEG findings of one sides temporal slowing

 

# Case 98

(see page 625 for Answers)

One day after being bitten on the leg by her cat, the parents of a 6-year-old girl note increased swelling and tenderness at the site. Her immunizations are up to date and the cat has scratched and bitten her before so the parents are surprised at how red this has gotten so fast.

## Question 1:

**The presentation is most likely due to:**

A) Idiopathic inflammation
B) *Bartonella henselae*
C) *Pasteurella multocida*
D) *Staph aureus*
E) *Strep Viridans*

## Question 2:

**Which of the following would be the most appropriate treatment?**

A) Warm soaks, no antibiotics
B) Amoxicillin-clavulanate
C) Dicloxacillin
D) Erythromycin
E) Clindamycin

## Question 3:

**Alternative treatments for *this* patient would include:**

A) Levofloxacin
B) Ampicillin
C) Doxycycline
D) Cephalexin
E) Cefadroxil

# Case 99

*(see page 629 for Answers)*

You are performing a routine physical examination on a full term newborn.

On physical examination you note a head circumference of 30 cm with a purpuric rash on the legs and arms. The abdomen is soft with marked hepatosplenomegaly.

CBC reveals a white blood cell count of 9.5 with a normal differential and a platelet count of 85, hematocrit of 36 and a hemoglobin of 12.
Bilirubin is 10.5/ 0.5

Ophthalmological consult confirms the presence of retinitis.

## Question 1:

**Which of the following diagnoses bests explains the patient's presentation?**

A) HIV
B) Henoch Schönlein purpura
C) Idiopathic thrombocytopenic purpura
D) Congenital CMV
E) Congenital toxoplasmosis

## Question 2:

**Which additional finding is likely to be discovered in this patient?**

A) Patent ductus arteriosis
B) Osteochondritis
C) Periventricular cerebral calcifications
D) Diffuse cerebral calcifications
E) Meningoencephalitis

# Case 100

(see page 631 for Answers)

You are evaluating a 4-month-old infant for a routine well baby visit. The baby has been feeding well and is developmentally normal. The baby is sleeping while you are taking a history from the mother and you notice a jugular pulse wave. You auscultate the heart and hear a soft murmur which is consistent with a flow murmur and a resting heart rate of 60.
You note that during previous physical exams the infant's heart rate is 80, 75, and 85.

By now the baby has woken up and is crying because he is hungry.
You listen to the heart rate again and it is 70.

## Question 1:

**Which of the following would be the most appropriate initial step in establishing a diagnosis?**

A) Recheck the heart rate on 3 separate occasions
B) Chest x-ray
C) Cardiac Echo
D) EKG
E) No studies are indicated

## Question 2:

**Which of the following is the most likely explanation for the child's presentation?**

A) VSD
B) BBC
C) Normal Findings
D) Congenital AV heart block
E) Acquired heart block

## Question 3:

**Which of the following might be necessary as a treatment modality?**

A) Surgical closure of the VSD
B) Eliminate any and all Podcasts® of the BBC
C) Eliminate the causative agent
D) Pacemaker
E) Jerry and the pacemakers

# Case 101

*(see page 633 for Answers)*

You are evaluating a 9-year-old girl with an acute onset of severe right-sided abdominal pain which is intermittent. She has been experiencing episodic vomiting. She has been afebrile with no diarrhea.

CBC shows a WBC 12.5 with a normal differential, electrolytes are within normal limits. Urinalysis is negative for blood, bacteria, and protein. Abdominal x-ray demonstrates some stool on the left side with no signs of obstruction. Abdominal and pelvic ultrasound reveals an echogenic intraovarian mass.

 

## Question 1:

**The most appropriate next step in managing this patient would be:**

A) CT with oral contrast
B) CT with oral and IV contrast
C) Doppler flow ultrasonography
D) Spiral CT without contrast
E) Overnight observation and pain management

## Question 2:

**The most likely diagnosis to explain the patient's condition would be:**

A) Acute appendicitis
B) Nephrolithiasis
C) Pyelonephritis
D) Ovarian Torsion
E) Constipation

## Question 3:

**The most appropriate management of this problem would be:**

A) Emergency Appendectomy
B) IV fluids and pain management
C) IV antibiotics
D) Laxatives and dietary counseling
E) Laparoscopic reversal of torsion

# Case 102

*(see page 635 for Answers)*

You are evaluating a 7-year-old girl who has been having difficulty walking unassisted. On physical exam you note some weakness of the arms which is less pronounced than the muscle weakness of the lower extremities.

The deep tendon reflexes are diminished in all 4 extremities. Sensory loss is limited to the face where you also note bilateral ptosis. There is no tenderness over the vertebral spine. The symptoms started late last night. Up until that point she has had no medical problems and her neurodevelopment has been normal and her immunizations are up to date.

 

## Question 1:

**The most likely explanation for the symptoms would be**

A) Neurological Tic
B) Tick bite
C) Guillain Barré
D) Myasthenia gravis
E) Acuter transverse myelitis

## Question 2:

**The most appropriate next step would be:**

A) Lumbar puncture
B) MRI of the spine
C) Tensilon Test
D) Diphenhydramine IV
E) Look for and remove all ticks

# Case 103

(see page 637 for Answers)

You are evaluating a 3-month-old infant on a routine followup visit. The infant is a former 29-week preemie who was in the NICU for several weeks and required mechanical ventilation for around 10 days. He has been diagnosed with bronchopulmonary dysplasia and has been treated with furosemide. A routine urine dipstick is positive for blood.

 

## Question 1:

**The most appropriate next step would be:**

A) Renal ultrasound
B) Urinalysis
C) Calcium: Creatinine ratio in a spot urine
D) 24-hour collection for urine calcium quantification
E) Abdominal CT scan

## Question 2:

**Each of the following will be helpful in working up this patient *except*:**

A) Serum calcium
B) Urine Calcium
C) Serum alkaline phosphatase
D) Serum phosphate
E) Serum creatinine

## Question 3:

**Which of the following is the most common cause of hypercalciuria in infants?**

A) Idiopathic hypercalciuria
B) Iatrogenic hypercalciuria
C) Wilms tumor
D) Bartter syndrome
E) Vitamin D toxicity

# Case 104

(see page 639 for Answers)

You are evaluating a 10-year-old girl who presents with a one-week history of crampy abdominal pain and malodorous diarrhea.

She has not travelled outside of the U.S. over the past year and has not gone camping. Her past history is negative except for a bout of pneumonia 6 weeks ago, which was successfully treated with a course of Azithromycin after a course of amoxicillin failed.

Physical examination is negative except for crampy abdominal pain.

She is in the 60th percentile for weight and height.

Stool sample is positive for the presence of white blood cells.

## Question 1:

**Which of the following would be the most appropriate initial study in this patient?**

A) String test for Giardia Lamblia
B) Serial stool testing for Entamoeba histolytica
C) Serum erythrocyte sedimentation rate
D) Stool culture for enteric pathogens
E) Stool sample for the presence of Clostridium difficile toxin.

## Question 2:

**Which of the following is the most likely diagnosis to explain the patient's presentation?**

A) Giardia lamblia enteritis
B) Amebiasis
C) Pseudomembranous colitis
D) Salmonella gastroenteritis
E) Inflammatory bowel disease

## Question 3:

**Which of the following would be the most appropriate treatment in this patient?**

A) Oral Metronidazole
B) IV Metronidazole
C) Systemic steroids
D) Barium Enema
E) Colonoscopy

# Case 105

(see page 641 for Answers)

You are evaluating an 8-year-old girl who has fallen behind in reading. She seems to have difficulty reading both at home and in school. You noticed her in the waiting room holding the magazine she was reading very close to her face. However the result of her vision check in your office is completely normal.

On physical exam her funduscopic exam is normal; pupils are equal and reactive to light. She sits in the front row where she is most comfortable and has no difficulty paying attention, gets along well with other children and is doing well in other subjects

 

## Question 1:

**The most likely diagnosis in this patient is:**

A) ADD without hyperactivity
B) ADHD
C) Mild mental retardation
D) Specific learning disability
E) Behavioral

## Question 2:

**The most appropriate intervention at this point would be:**

A) Atomoxetine
B) Methylphenidate
C) Ophthalmology referral
D) Cognitive testing
E) Token behavioral modification

## Question 3:

**The most common ophthalmological problem in children is:**

A) Myopia
B) Hyperopia
C) Esotropia
D) Exotropia
E) Pseudoesotropia

# Case 106

*(see page 643 for Answers)*

You are evaluating a 3-year-old boy who has had a severe gastroenteritis for the past four days. Initially he was vomiting with watery diarrhea. Over the past day and a half the diarrhea has continued but he was able to hold down fluids and has been given water and apple juice which he has been tolerating well.

Despite this, he is lethargic with muscle aches, a heart rate of 115, respiratory rate of 25, and temperature of 100.3F. His capillary refill is less than 2 seconds, his mucous membranes are moist and he has good tear production. His abdominal exam is benign with no guarding or rebound tenderness. He has urinated twice today.

 

## Question 1:

**The most likely explanation for this patient's presentation is:**

A) Hypokalemia
B) Hyperkalemia
C) Hyperglycemia
D) Hypernatremic dehydration
E) Severe dehydration

## Question 2:

**Which of the following would be of immediate concern in this patient?**

A) Life-threatening arrhythmias
B) Cerebral edema
C) Pontine myelinolysis
D) SIADH
E) Metabolic acidosis

## Question 3:

**The most important step in *initially* managing this patient would be:**

A) 12-lead EKG
B) Potassium bolus (0.3 mEq / Kg)
C) Potassium chloride infusion
(1MeQ / Kg/ hour)
D) Sodium bolus (0.3meQ/Kg)
E) Normal Saline Bolus (20 ml/Kg)

# Case 107

(see page 645 for Answers)

You are evaluating a 6-week-old male infant diagnosed with colic who now presents with large loose stools that contain bloody streaks. The mother initially breast fed for the first 4 weeks of life and started a standard infant formula upon returning to work.

On physical examination the infant is afebrile with normal vital signs. Abdomen is soft with normal bowel sounds.
The stool pH is 5.30.

 

## Question 1:

**The most likely explanation for the loose stools would be:**

A) Anal fissure
B) Giardiasis
C) Galactosemia
D) Cow milk protein intolerance
E) Intussusception

## Question 2:

**The most appropriate initial management for this patient would be:**

A) Soy formula
B) Metronidazole
C) Galactose free diet
D) Air contrast enema
E) Protein hydrolysate formula

# Case 108

(see page 647 for Answers)

A 6-month-old infant with Down syndrome is brought to you by his parents because of an intermittent history of episodes where his hands and feet turn blue. The rest of the time his hands and feet have a mottled appearance. He has been gaining weight steadily and on physical examination there is no murmur and the infant is not tachypneic nor in any distress while feeding. EKG is within normal limits for age and chest x-ray shows no cardiomegaly and normal pulmonary vascularity.

 

## Question 1:

**Which of the following would be the most appropriate next step in this infant?**

A) Reassurance
B) Cardiac echo
C) Pulse oximetry
D) Cardiac catheterization
E) Chest CT

## Question 2:

**The most likely diagnosis in this patient would be:**

A) Eisenmenger syndrome
B) AV septal defect
C) VSD
D) Muchos cutis muchachos
E) Cutis marmorata physiologica

## Question 3:

**Children with Down syndrome are at increased risk for each of the following *except*:**

A) Poor weight gain
B) Decreased pulmonary vascular resistance
C) AV septal defects
D) Right ventricular hypertrophy
E) Left to right shunting

# Case 109

*(see page 651 for Answers)*

You are called to the delivery room to evaluate an infant who is apneic. The infant was delivered by elective repeat C/Section. There was no meconium staining. The delivery room staff has suctioned out the nasopharynx and found no meconium. They have been providing bag mask ventilation and you notice that the chest wall is not expanding and the infant appears to be cyanotic. You step in to take over the resuscitation.

## Question 1:

**After suctioning out the airway your next step in resuscitating this baby would be:**

A) Continue bag mask ventilation with increased pressures
B) Endotracheal intubation to establish an airway
C) Endotracheal intubation and epinephrine via the ET tube
D) Take over bag mask ventilation and have an assistant begin chest compressions
E) Discontinue bag mask ventilation for a trial of tactile stimulation

## Question 2:

**Once stabilized the most likely diagnosis will be:**

A) Transient tachypnea of the newborn
B) Congenital heart disease
C) Meconium aspiration
D) Primary pulmonary hypertension
E) Hyaline membrane disease

# Case 110

*(see page 653 for Answers)*

A 14-year-old boy has been experiencing difficulty holding objects in the morning especially when he has not gotten adequate sleep. He has similar difficulty holding other objects in the morning and occasionally has odd jerky movements of his arms that he cannot control. In the past he has been diagnosed with absence seizures but he is no longer receiving treatment. He has had no absence seizures for several years.

A recent EEG result shows bilateral 3 to 6 cycles per second polyspike and wave discharges.

## Question 1:

**What of the following diagnoses explains the patient's presentation?**

A) Pseudoseizure
B) Absence seizure variation
C) Idiopathic tics
D) Juvenile myoclonic epilepsy
E) Rolandic Seizures

## Question 2:

**The best treatment for this disorder is:**

A) Haloperidol
B) Valproic acid
C) Risperidone
D) Methylphenidate
E) Supportive care only

## Question 3:

**The likelihood of the condition resolving and not requiring medical treatment is closest to:**

A) 0%
B) 25%
C) 50 %
D) 75%
E) 100%

# Case 111

(see page 655 for Answers)

You are evaluating a 10-year-old girl who has been experiencing intermittent diurnal urinary incontinence. She has previously been fully continent. She has been afebrile, experienced no dysuria, and is afebrile in your office.

On physical exam there is no suprapubic tenderness and vaginal exam is unremarkable. Urinalysis is negative for blood, protein, leukocyte esterase and nitrites. Urine glucose is negative. A Urine culture grew out no organisms and spot urine revealed calcium: creatinine ratio of 0.12 (less than 0.2 is normal). She has otherwise been healthy with no prior illnesses or surgery.

 

## Question 1:

**The most appropriate next step in this patient would be:**

A) Reassurance and management
B) Renal ultrasound
C) VCUG
D) 24 hour urine calcium quantification
E) Abdominal and pelvic ultrasound

## Question 2:

**The most likely diagnosis to explain this patient's presentation would be?**

A) Unstable bladder
B) Grade 1 vesicoureteral reflux
C) Grade 5 vesicoureteral reflux
D) Hypercalciuria
E) Hinman syndrome

## Question 3:

**The most appropriate management would be:**

A) Anticholinergic medication
B) Intermittent antibiotics
C) Surgical correction
D) Hydrochlorothiazide
E) Intermittent catheterization

 

# Case 112

(see page 657 for Answers)

You are evaluating an infant at his 2-week followup. The infant was born by normal spontaneous vaginal birth, and has done well up until recently when the mother noticed that he has been breathing fast and has decreased the frequency of and duration of feedings. In addition he appears to be sweating a lot.

On physical examination you note that the baby is breathing greater than 75 per minute with nasal flaring. Peripheral pulses are weak especially in the lower extremity. On auscultation you note a gallop rhythm.

 

## Question 1:

**The most likely underlying cause of the infant's presentation is:**

A) Tetralogy of Fallot
B) Choanal atresia
C) Gastroesophageal reflux
D) Transposition of the great vessels
E) Coarctation of the aorta

## Question 2:

**Which of the following would best establish the correct diagnosis?**

A) Head CT
B) pH probe study
C) Cardiac Echo
D) EKG
E) Cardiac catheterization

## Question 3:

**The most appropriate *initial* treatment would consist of :**

A) NG feedings
B) Histamine blocking medications
C) Prostaglandin E
D) IV antibiotics
E) Endotracheal intubation

 

# Case 113

*(see page 659 for Answers)*

A 2-year-old is brought to your office because of a peculiar rash brought to the parent's attention by the nurse at the day care center the child attends. The child is afebrile and other wise doing well with no prior history of pneumonia, recurrent otitis media or epistaxis.

On physical examination the child is afebrile and you note a scaly rash on the scalp especially in front of the ears with a similar pattern in the underarms and diaper area. You note that the rash consists of several small lesions measuring 2-4 mm, which are erythematous brownish papules with some petechiae. Skin biopsy reveals monocyte macrophages containing Birbeck's granules.

## Question 1:

**Which of the following primary disorders is the most likely diagnosis to explain this patient's presentation?**

A) Class I Histiocytosis
B) Class III Histiocytosis
C) Wiskott Aldrich Syndrome
D) Psoriasis
E) Acrodermatitis enterohepatica

## Question 2:

**Each of the following *specific* clinical entities would be included in the differential diagnosis for this patient *except*:**

A) Hand Schüller-Christian disease
B) Eosinophilic granuloma
C) Malignant histiocytosis
D) Letter Siwe Disease
E) Langerhans Cell histiocytosis

# Case 114

*(see page 663 for Answers)*

You are evaluating a newborn at 2 weeks and note that there is difficulty with abduction of the hips. The gluteal folds, however, are symmetrical. You suspect bilateral subluxation on physical examination.

## Question 1:

**Which of the following is true regarding making the correct diagnosis in this patient?**

A) Ortolani test is diagnostic
B) Barlow test is diagnostic
C) Plain x-ray is diagnostic
D) Ultrasound is diagnostic
E) Diagnosis isn't definitive until 2 months of age

## Question 2:

**Which of the following is true regarding developmental dysplasia of the hip?**

A) It is more common among females
B) It is more common among males
C) It is more prevalent among African American newborns
D) It occurs more frequently on the right side
E) Asymmetric gluteal folds is a specific sign

## Question 3:

**Which of the following is true regarding management of developmental dysplasia of the hip?**

A) Treatment success is confirmed on ultrasound
B) Double diapers are sufficient to treat most cases
C) The Pavlik harness is the standard treatment
D) Non surgical management must be done before 12 months
E) Findings are always evident at birth

 

# Case 115

(see page 665 for Answers)

You are evaluating an 8-month-old infant who has been distressed over the past 2 hours and unable to feed. You evaluate the infant and note that he is diaphoretic, pale and in significant distress and inconsolable. On physical examination the infant is afebrile with a respiratory rate of 50 breaths per minute but you have a difficult time obtaining a peripheral pulse.
You place the infant on a monitor and note a heart rate of 250 with narrow complexes.
Prior to this, the infant's growth and development were within normal limits.

 

## Question 1:

**The most likely explanation for the child's presentation:**

A) Congestive heart failure
B) Ventricular septal defect
C) Congenital hyperthyroidism
D) Graves disease
E) Supraventricular tachycardia

## Question 2:

**After administering oxygen the most appropriate next step in managing this baby would be:**

A) IV propranolol
B) Facial ice compress
C) Verapamil IV push
D) Adenosine IV slow push
E) Adenosine IV rapid push followed by normal saline flush

# Case 116

(see page 667 for Answers)

You are "taking a break" working as a camp doctor and you are holding your weekly clinic just before going bass fishing. A 12-year-old boy appears from *his* bass fishing trip[1] wearing short pants and a tank top shirt. You, on the other hand, are wearing scrub cutoffs and a tank top lab coat despite the fact that your narcissistic lack of awareness is causing humiliating embarrassment for your children who are also attending the camp. He (we're back to the patient now) has gone fishing everyday for a week, and has developed a worsening rash over the past 2 days.

The rash appears on his arms and legs sparing his trunk, groin area, face and scalp. The rash is linear and pruritic with erythematous papules and vesicles.

1 He lets you know the fishing was fantastic all morning but now nothing for the past two hours, pouring cold water on your hopes to catch anything.

 

## Question 1:

**The most likely diagnosis would be:**

A) Scabies
B) Ichthyosis
C) Erysipelas
D) Atopic dermatitis
E) Contact dermatitis

## Question 2:

**The most appropriate treatment would be:**

A) Lindane 1%
B) Permethrin 5%
C) Topical corticosteroid
D) Prednisone
E) Cephalexin

## Question 3:

**The rash would best be characterized as a:**

A) Type 1 allergic reaction
B) Type 2 allergic reaction
C) Type 3 allergic reaction
D) Type 4 allergic reaction
E) Not my type reaction

# Case 117

(see page 669 for Answers)

A 26-month-old boy in your practice presents with a history of vomiting and severe abdominal pain. In addition the parents have brought along a diaper containing bloody stools. The pain is severe and then will sometimes stop suddenly. He was seen in your office last week for an upper respiratory tract infection. The boy is afebrile

He was initially sleeping and the parents asked that you hold off on examining him since he has not gotten much rest in the past 24 hours. You gently palpate the abdomen and note no tenderness, guarding or rebound.

They call you back into the room 15 minutes later. The child is now squirming and screaming in extreme pain. The abdomen is now tender with marked guarding. You are unable to assess for rebound tenderness due to the severity of the pain.

## Question 1:

**The most appropriate next step in managing this patient would be:**

A) Abdominal CT with IV contrast
B) Abdominal CT with Oral and IV contrast.
C) Serum CBC, electrolytes and Stool culture for enteric pathogens
D) Abdominal ultrasound
E) Air contrast enema

## Question 2:

**The most likely diagnosis would be:**

A) Inflammatory bowel disease
B) Acute appendicitis
C) Acute pancreatitis
D) Intussusception
E) Yersinia gastroenteritis

## Question 3:

**The most effective treatment for this patient would be:**

A) Colonoscopy
B) Surgical excision
C) IV antibiotics and pain control
D) Air contrast enema
E) Oral antibiotics

 

# Case 118

*(see page 671 for Answers)*

You are evaluating a 12-year-old boy who, up until this point, has been healthy, in fact, quite athletic. He presents this morning with weakness of the entire left side of his body. His cognition and speech are within normal limits as are his hearing and vision.

On physical exam you note marked motor weakness of his left lower and upper extremities and marked tenderness over his chest where you note ecchymoses. The patient then recalls getting hit in the chest by a rushing opponent yesterday who knocked the wind out of the patient but he was able to finish the game. There was no loss of consciousness and he denies getting hit on the head at all.

 

## Question 1:

**The most appropriate study to order to identify the cause of the patient's symptoms would be:**

A) Head CT
B) Head MRI
C) Chest CT
D) Carotid Angiography
E) Head MRA

## Question 2:

**The most likely etiology for this patient's presentation would be:**

A) Subdural hematoma
B) Epidural hematoma
C) Basilar skull fracture
D) Vertebral fracture
E) Embolic stroke

# Case 119

*(see page 673 for Answers)*

You are evaluating a 14-year-old boy brought in by EMS to the pediatric ER. He was found passed out in the back yard by his friends. You are unable to arouse him although he does respond to painful stimuli. His pupils are miotic but equal and reactive. His temperature is 97.8 F; respiratory rate is 10 with a shallow breathing pattern. His heart rate is 55 and blood pressure is 95/65.

 

## Question 1:

**The most likely diagnosis to explain the patient's presentation would be:**

A) Septic shock
B) Alcohol ingestion
C) Organophosphate toxicity
D) Opiate overdose
E) PCP overdose

## Question 2:

**The most appropriate initial step in managing this patient is:**

A) Look up the word miotic
B) Intramuscular naloxone
C) IV normal Saline bolus
D) Endotracheal intubation
E) Chest compressions

## Question 3:

**Once stabilized the most appropriate management would be:**

A) Thiamine IM
B) IV Glucose bolus
C) IV Normal Saline
D) IM naloxone
E) IV Atropine

# Case 120

*(see page 675 for Answers)*

You are evaluating a 15-month-old boy who has been vomiting for 48 hours with copious watery diarrhea.
He has had no wet diapers today.
On physical exam the toddler is very ill appearing and listless, with a temperature of 101.2, heart rate of 180. Abdominal exam is remarkable for doughy skin with no guarding or rebound tenderness. Capillary refill is greater than 3 seconds.

 

## Question 1:

**The degree of dehydration in this patient can best be characterized as:**

A) Mild
B) Moderate
C) Severe
D) Dry
E) Halloween wicked

## Question 2:

**The type of dehydration can best be categorized as:**

A) Hyponatremic
B) Hypernatremic
C) Isotonic
D) Hypokalemic
E) Electrostatic and Enigmatic

# Case 121

(see page 677 for Answers)

An 18-month-old child in your practice has been observed by his parents and baby-sitter eating dirt on numerous occasions. His growth and development are normal. His immunizations are up to date and his height and weight are at the 60th percentile for age. His nutrition is appropriate for age.

On physical examination the child is afebrile, TMs intact, funduscopic exam is unremarkable. His abdomen is soft with hepatosplenomegaly.

His screening CBC shows a WBC of 12.5. Hematocrit is 38 with hemoglobin of 12.5, 10% neutrophils 10 % lymphocytes and 80% eosinophils, platelet count of 175.

 

## Question 1:

**The most likely diagnosis would be:**

A) Chronic Asthma
B) Enterobius vermicularis
C) Visceral larva migrans
D) Toxocara canis
E) Plumbism

## Question 2:

**The most appropriate test to establish the diagnosis would be:**

A) Pulmonary function testing
B) Scotch tape test
C) Stool for ova and parasites
D) Serological testing
E) Serum lead levels

## Question 3:

**The most appropriate treatment would be:**

A) Albuterol
B) Albendazole
C) Iron supplementation
D) IV chelation
E) Improved hygiene

# Case 122

(see page 679 for Answers)

You are assigned a full-term newborn born to a 35-year-old multigravida recent immigrant from Guatemala. The infant had an indirect bilirubin level of 12.1 and direct of 0.4 at 6 hours of age, which is now 19.4/0.4– the baby has had stool production

The mother is O negative and the baby is B positive. The infant on exam is icteric with a soft abdomen, no hepatomegaly. Heart S1, S2 no murmur, with normal retinal exam with good red reflex. The baby is alert and responsive. Other than mild cephalohematoma the baby is normocephalic with no abnormalities noted.

## Question 1:

**The most likely explanation for the infant's hyperbilirubinemia is:**

A) Physiologic jaundice
B) Cytomegalovirus infection
C) Hemolysis
D) B: O incompatibility
E) Rh incompatibility

## Question 2:

**The most important immediate intervention:**

A) Suspend breast feeding for 48 hours
B) Culture for cytomegalovirus
C) Soy formula
D) Phototherapy and hydration
E) Liver ultrasound

# Case 123

*(see page 681 for Answers)*

A 16-year-old girl presents with an erythematous rash on her cheeks and nasal area. In addition she has a rash on her hands which is also erythematous, scaly and limited to the dorsal aspect of her hands in between the joints. The patient has been experiencing thinning hair and hair loss.
On physical examination the patient experiences sharp chest pain with inspiration.

 

## Question 1:

**Which of the following would be most helpful in establishing the correct diagnosis?**

A) Serum ANA
B) Serum Antibody to SM nuclear antigen
C) Serum creatinine kinase
D) Muscle biopsy
E) Rheumatoid factor

## Question 2:

**Which of the following can be seen in patients with this condition?**

A) False positive VDRL
B) False positive FTA-ABS
C) Gottron papules
D) Heliotropic rash
E) Positive Gowers maneuver

# Case 124

*(see page 683 for Answers)*

A 12-year-old boy presents with a circular violaceous rash which, when palpated, feels like there are firm papules underneath.
He was treated with topical nystatin for 10 days followed by a ten-day course of clotrimazole with no clinical improvement.

 

## Question 1:

**The most likely diagnosis is :**

A) Nummular Eczema
B) Erythema multiforme
C) Tinea Corporis
D) Erysipelas
E) Granuloma annulare

## Question 2:

**The most appropriate treatment would be:**

A) Higher potency anti-fungal cream
B) Immediate admission to a burn unit
C) Oral Antifungal agents
D) Topical Mupirocin
E) Reassurance that this will resolve spontaneously

# Case 125

(see page 685 for Answers)

You are evaluating a 16-year-old girl with a 7 week history of mild anxiety and increased heart rate evaluated at the local ER and dismissed as pre exam jitters with a normal EKG; she has lost 7 pounds in the past month. You ask her about her weight and she tells you that she is okay with it but is concerned about the weight she lost.

On physical exam she is afebrile, somewhat anxious but appropriate. Her heart rate is 110 with a respiratory rate of 18 and blood pressure of 135/85. Cap refill is less than 2 seconds with 2 + pulses throughout. You note a soft systolic ejection murmur heard best on the left side. Her abdomen is soft with no hepatomegaly. Lungs are clear. EKG reveals a sinus tachycardia with a normal p wave preceding each QRS complex of normal width.

 

## Question 1:

**The most likely diagnosis to explain the patient's presentation would be**

A) Panic attack
B) Anorexia nervosa
C) Supraventricular tachycardia
D) Hyperthyroidism
E) Wolf Parkinson White syndrome

## Question 2:

**The most appropriate initial diagnostic step would be**

A) Thyroid Scan
B) Thyroid Stimulation hormone level
C) Cardiac Echo
D) IV adenosine via rapid infusion
E) Urine toxicology screen

# Case 126

*(see page 687 for Answers)*

You are evaluating a 5-month-old infant who, up until 3 weeks ago, was growing normally and doing fine. Over the past few weeks he has become increasingly tachypneic and has not gained any weight. Physical exam reveals a respiratory rate of 75 and grade 2 systolic ejection murmur with no signs of cyanosis. The EKG is normal and the chest x-ray reveals increased vascularity with no cardiomegaly.

## Question 1:

**The most likely explanation for the child's presentation would be:**

A) Intracranial arteriovenous malformation
B) Intraabdominal arteriovenous malformation
C) Hypoplastic left heart syndrome
D) Transposition of the great vessels
E) Supracardiac total anomalous venous return

## Question 2:

**The primary reason for the presenting symptoms would be:**

A) Right to left shunting of blood across the foramen ovale
B) Left to right shunting of blood across the foramen ovale
C) Poor left ventricular ejection fraction
D) Increased right sided pre-load
E) Increased systemic resistance

 

# Case 127

(see page 689 for Answers)

A 6-year-old presents with a rash that has developed over the past two months. The rash is seen on the extensor surface of the knees, they eyebrows and behind the ears. On physical exam you note erythematous raised plaques. On the extensor surface of the elbows you note pinpoint areas of hemorrhaging.

## Question 1:

**The most likely diagnosis to explain the findings in this patient would be:**

A) Nummular Eczema
B) Psoriasis
C) Tinea corpus
D) Atopic dermatitis
E) Bullous impetigo

## Question 2:

**The best initial treatment for this patient would be:**

A) Topical antifungal cream
B) Oral antifungal medication
C) Topical steroids
D) Oral steroids
E) Emollients

## Question 3:

**Which of the following can be an associated finding?**

A) Chronic antibiotic use
B) Asthma
C) Post strep glomerulonephritis
D) Deficiency in zinc transport
E) Koebner phenomenon

# Case 128

*(see page 691 for Answers)*

A 2-year-old boy presents with a recurrent rash that is best described as scaling patches which are erythematous and concentrated on the upper and lower extremities, face and the scalp with sparing of the diaper area.

The boy has been hospitalized 3 times for lobar pneumonia; during one episode blood cultures grew out *Streptococcus pneumoniae*. He also has experienced recurrent epistaxis.
On CBC he has a WBC of 12.5 with a normal differential. Hematocrit is 38 and his platelet count is 40 thousand.

## Question 1:

**The most likely explanation for this patient's presentation would be:**

A) Idiopathic thrombocytopenic purpura
B) Histiocytosis Type 1
C) Histiocytosis Type 2
D) Acrodermatitis enteropathica
E) Wiskott Aldrich Syndrome

## Question 2:

**Which of the following is also seen in patients with this disorder?**

A) Splenomegaly
B) Birbeck granules
C) Atopic dermatitis
D) Vitiligo
E) Reactive Airway disease

## Question 3:

**Which of the following best describes the primary inheritance pattern of this disorder?**

A) Autosomal dominant
B) Autosomal recessive
C) X- Linked recessive
D) X- Linked dominant
E) Random mutation

# Case 129

*(see page 693 for Answers)*

A 4-year-old girl returns from a trip to Long Island to visit her grandparents and presents with fever, muscles aches, shaking chills and headache.
Three days later you note a petechial rash on the wrists and ankles.
Her immunizations are up to date.

On physical exam the child is low in energy and cranky and has a temperature of 102.

 

## Question 1:

**The most likely explanation for this child's symptoms is:**

A) Sleep deprived exhaustion
B) Lyme disease
C) Rocky Mountain spotted fever
D) Meningococcemia
E) Measles

## Question 2:

**The most appropriate study to perform in this patient is:**

A) Sleep study
B) Lyme titers
C) Rickettsia rickettsii titers
D) Rubeola titers
E) Implement treatment only

## Question 3:

**The most appropriate treatment in this patient would be:**

A) Doxycycline
B) Chloramphenicol
C) Ceftriaxone
D) Ampicillin
E) Oral Amoxicillin for 21 days

 

# Case 130

(see page 695 for Answers)

You are caring for a 15-year-old boy who presents with severe headache, runny nose, sore throat and a temperature of 101.2 F. A cough that started 3 days ago has gotten much worse to the point that his voice is hoarse. Auscultation of his chest is significant for rales and wheezes throughout the lung fields. You order a chest x-ray that reveals bilateral interstitial infiltrates concentrated in the lower lobes.

All of his immunizations are up to date and he has not done any recent travel.

## Question 1:

**Which of the following studies would be most helpful in establishing the correct diagnosis?**

A) Serological testing for *Mycoplasma pneumoniae*
B) Serum cold hemagglutinin levels
C) RSV antigen testing
D) Culture of sputum
E) Throat culture for Group A beta hemolytic strep

## Question 2:

**Which of the following is the most likely diagnosis?**

A) Aspergillosis
B) Histoplasmosis
C) RSV pneumonia
D) *Mycoplasma pneumonia*
E) Pertussis

## Question 3:

**Which of the following best describes the primary inheritance pattern of this disorder?**

A) IV Amphotericin B
B) Supportive care and isolation
C) Amoxicillin
D) Augmentin
E) Azithromycin

 

# Case 131

*(see page 697 for Answers)*

You are evaluating a newborn on day two of life who has been experiencing clonic seizures which have been observed independently by 3 nurses. You have been called to observe an episode which you note lasting 120 seconds involving the hands and left leg. The Apgars were 8 and 9 and the delivery was a spontaneous vaginal delivery although vacuum extraction was required.
The CBC and electrolytes are within normal limits.
Bilirubin 1/0.5 total and direct.

A lumbar puncture is done with the following results:

Marked xanthochromia with RBC 1200/cubic millimeter
Protein 600 mg/dL

 

## Question 1:

**The most appropriate next step in establishing a diagnosis would be:**

A) Repeat lumbar puncture
B) Head ultrasound
C) Head CT
D) Head MRI
E) EEG

## Question 2:

**The most likely explanation for the clonic seizures in this infant would be:**

A) Kernicterus
B) Ischemic encephalopathy
C) Subarachnoid hemorrhage
D) Subdural hemorrhage
E) Meningitis

## Question 3:

**This patient will most likely require:**

A) Phototherapy
B) Subdural tap
C) Serial head circumference evaluation
D) IV acyclovir
E) IV Ampicillin/Cefotaxime

# Case 132

(see page 699 for Answers)

You are evaluating a newborn who has had wheezing present since birth. The wheezing is worse whenever the child is feeding or crying. The mother also notes that the wheezing gets worse whenever the infant's neck is flexed. A right-sided aortic arch is noted on chest x-ray.

## Question 1:

**The most likely diagnosis in this patient would be:**

A) Meconium aspiration
B) Gastroesophageal reflux
C) Vascular ring
D) Bronchiolitis
E) Tracheoesophageal fistula

## Question 2:

**Additional steps in managing this patient should include:**

A) Sweat Test
B) Home apnea monitoring
C) Barium Swallow
D) Chest x-ray following placement of ET Tube
E) pH probe study

# Case 133

*(see page 701 for Answers)*

A 2-1/2 year old toddler was found with an opened bottle of his grandmother's imipramine pills. They are not sure how many pills were in the bottle and there were some contents found on the toddler's mouth and tongue. On physical exam the toddler is alert and responsive, afebrile and vital signs stable.

## Question 1:

**The child would be at risk for each of the following *except*:**

A) Hypertension
B) Hypotension
C) Cardiac arrest
D) S-T shifts
E) Miosis

## Question 2:

**Which of the following would be the most appropriate immediate management?**

A) Syrup of Ipecac
B) Activated charcoal with sorbitol
C) Activated charcoal
D) Nasogastric lavage with normal saline
E) Endotracheal intubation to protect airway

## Question 3:

**Which of the following would be *most helpful* in assessing this child?**

A) Serum electrolytes
B) Baseline Chest x-ray
C) Baseline EKG
D) Salicylate and Acetaminophen levels
E) Liver function studies

# Case 134

(see page 703 for Answers)

You are evaluating a 2-day-old newborn who presents with bilateral leukocoria and routine hearing screening suggests sensorineural hearing loss.
You also note facial purpura lesions and hepatosplenomegaly.

## Question 1:

**The most likely explanation for these findings would be:**

A) Congenital rubella
B) Meningococcemia
C) Toxoplasmosis
D) Congenital CMV
E) Disseminated herpes simplex virus

## Question 2:

**Another finding associated with this disease would be:**

A) Pulmonary artery stenosis
B) Keratitis
C) Chorioretinitis
D) Thrombocytosis
E) Temporal lobe seizures

 

# Case 135

(see page 705 for Answers)

You are evaluating a 3-year-old child with a chronic rash described as dry, scaly patches concentrated on the extensor surfaces and the face since infancy. He now presents with oozing crusting lesions that are not scaly as previous lesions were and are not responding to previous treatments which, in the past, have been successful.

## Question 1:

**Which of the following diagnoses would explain the current presentation?**

A) Atopic dermatitis
B) Bullous impetigo
C) Histiocytosis Type I
D) Wiskott Aldrich Syndrome
E) Psoriasis

## Question 2:

**Which of the following would be most appropriate for this patient?**

A) Topical antibiotic cream
B) Oral antibiotics
C) Low potency topical steroids
D) Medium potency topical steroid
E) High Potency topical steroid cream

# Answers Section

# Case 1

(see page 3 for Questions)

History consistent with a diagnosis of dyslexia

A 9-year-old boy, although very popular with other students, is brought to your office by his parents because of some concerns expressed by his teacher. One example was a book report that was based on the book's illustrations but had no relation to the actual text. He has no difficulty understanding abstract concepts but has a difficult time completing exams that require written explanations. In addition, his handwriting is difficult to decipher. The family denies any extraordinary tension at home and there are no emotional difficulties at school or at home that the parents know about.

Rules out a low IQ or other cognitive deficits. This would also point away from a diagnosis of ADHD

This points away from depression or other endogenous or exogenous emotional difficulties or mood disorders.

## Question 1:

C) Phonemic awareness

## Question 2:

E) More time to take tests

The child in the vignette is displaying some classic signs of dyslexia. Handing in a book report that is based on the illustrations in the book rather than the text is consistent with a child with difficulty in reading comprehension (but too proud to admit it). Poor handwriting would be consistent with both dyslexia and ADHD but the ability to focus and grasp abstract concepts and explain these to others belies a diagnosis of ADHD. Similarly, this also points away from a low IQ as an explanation.

Dyslexia is a deficit in *phonemic awareness.* In case you were wondering what this is here is the explanation:

A phoneme is the "smallest discernible segment of speech", which in plain English is the sounds that are the components of words. These are even smaller than syllables; for example Pet would be "P" , "ae" and "t". (Remember "Hooked on Phonics®"?) Being aware of these sounds is what "phonemic awareness" is about and this is deficient in children with dyslexia.

Dyslexia is the most common learning disorder. The most effective intervention for children with dyslexia is to allow them more time to take tests. This is an example of accommodation. Remediation by working on phonemes and reading skills are usually less useful as the child ages.

 

# Case 2

(see page 5 for Questions)

Age and presentations are consistent with the diagnosis of ADHD

An 11-year-old boy in your practice has been having increasing difficulty paying attention in class. In addition to forgetting to take home and complete his homework assignments on time he frequently fidgets in class and talks out of turn. He was diagnosed with ADHD and started on long-acting methylphenidate, which resulted in dramatic improvement in his ability to stay focused at class and at home as evidenced by his turning in his homework assignments on a regular basis.

Patient experienced significant improvement on methylphenidate

Over the past few weeks he has been experiencing intermittent facial twitching as well as throat clearing. These increase when he is anxious and at the end of the day when he is most tired.

Tics

 

## Question 1:

E) Continue methylphenidate

## Question 2:

E) Dopamine receptor antagonists

## Question 3:

D) Premonitory urges preceding often represent greater morbidity than the tic itself

While the initiation of methylphenidate may *correlate with* an increase in tics it is usually transient and rarely worsens with methylphenidate treatment. It is also important to note that up to 50% of children with Tourette syndrome also have ADHD, with the symptoms of ADHD usually preceding the symptoms of Tourette syndrome.

This is why it was once believed that stimulant medication *caused the tics.* However a recent study by the Tourette syndrome study group provided solid evidence that to avoid methylphenidate because of worsening tics is unsubstantiated. Thus, with this patient the most appropriate step to take is to continue methylphenidate.

Alpha-2-adrenergic agonists would be appropriate for treating a primary tic disorder but not a patient who also has ADHD and has improved with methylphenidate. Therefore the correct answer to Question 1 is to continue treating with methylphenidate.

As note above methylphenidate has not be been proven to cause tic disorders. Of the medications listed the only ones known to actually cause a movement disorder are dopamine antagonist medications, the neuroleptic antipsychotic medications that can cause acute dystonic reactions or permanent movement disorders such as tardive dyskinesia.

Tourette syndrome is the 2nd most common primary tic disorder; the most common is "transient tic disorder". The recommended initial treatment for tics is *alpha-2 adrenergic agents such as clonidine* and *guanfacine.*

Premonitory urges can often cause severe anxiety especially in older children so much so that the morbidity associated with these urges is often worse than the tic itself. Therefore, voluntary suppression would not be a useful strategy for the management of tics, as it only increases anxiety and tension.

# Case 3

(see page 9 for Questions)

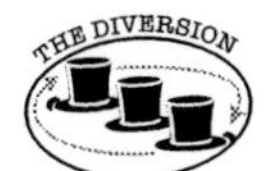


This implies pyloric stenosis as a diagnosis. However, the parents noting that the vomiting is forceful in quotes means it is not necessarily projectile vomiting

You are asked to evaluate a 2-month-old boy who had 2 episodes of vomiting over the past 4 days. The vomiting is non-bilious and "forceful" according to the parents. He is afebrile and his vital signs are stable. He is not feeding well and has been quite irritable. You attempt to feed the baby and notice that the baby arches backward while feeding and you decide to keep the baby in your office to observe while the parents attempt to feed.

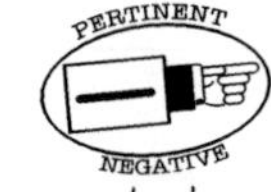


Afebrile, rules out meningitis

Very non-specific and not very helpful

Arching of the back is also consistent with an acute dystonic reaction (in addition to GERD)

Reglan® is one of the medications that causes an acute dystonic reaction and is an important part of the history.

His regular pediatrician has diagnosed GERD and started treatment with ranitidine and 2 days ago, when the vomiting progressed, added Reglan® (metoclopramide) which did not improve the symptoms

*(Continued on next page)*

*(Continued from previous page)*

at all. In fact the parents noted similar arching behavior and the "weird movements" you saw in the office. They just thought the baby was tired. His past history is unremarkable and his immunizations are up to date.

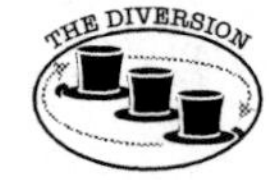


Here they are trying to divert you into believing you are dealing with a classic epileptic seizure but the rest of the story goes against a diagnosis of epilepsy.

A half-hour after trying to feed the baby, he becomes stiff, and clenches his fists with his eyes deviated to the right. He does not respond to tactile stimulation during this episode but there is no color change noted.

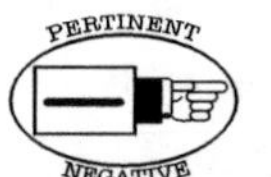


Since it does not respond to rectal diazepam this suggests a diagnosis other than seizures.

After establishing that the baby's vital signs are stable you provide diazepam rectally but the movements continue.

## Question 1:

C) IV diphenhydramine

## Question 2:

E) Acute dystonic reaction

## Question 3:

B) Discontinue metoclopramide

The correct diagnosis is an *acute dystonic reaction to metoclopramide.*

At first glance this patient's presentation is confusing and it is easy to Crosswire with other possibilities in the differential. However the lack of response to diazepam, the negative history and the presentation points away from a diagnosis of epilepsy.

While Sandifer syndrome can present with dystonia of the head and neck in conjunction with a history of GERD, one would expect symptoms to improve with treatment with metoclopramide rather than worsen.

The most appropriate immediate treatment would be diphenhydramine. If you picked promethazine you should actually lose points since this is a medication that can trigger an acute dystonic reaction. IV diazepam wouldn't be any more effective than PR and lorazepam is in the same class and unlikely to help. Benztropine is inappropriate for a child this young

Long-term outcome would be achieved by discontinuing the offending agent, in this case, metoclopramide.

# Case 4

(see page 13 for Questions)

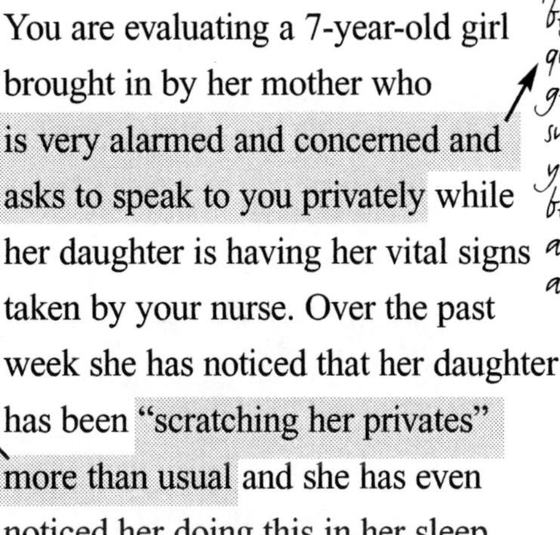
You are evaluating a 7-year-old girl brought in by her mother who is very alarmed and concerned and asks to speak to you privately while her daughter is having her vital signs taken by your nurse. Over the past week she has noticed that her daughter has been "scratching her privates" more than usual and she has even noticed her doing this in her sleep.

Yesterday she noticed that her daughter was somewhat irritable and had discovered blood on her panties although she did fall on a chair during recess. She also has had bouts of constipation recently. Her past medical history is negative except for a couple of nosebleeds last winter.

(Continued on next page)

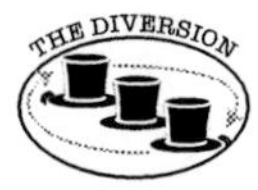


*The mother's alarm placed right at the beginning of the question is there to get your alarm and suspicions up so that you, too, are lead to believe that this is all due to sexual abuse.*

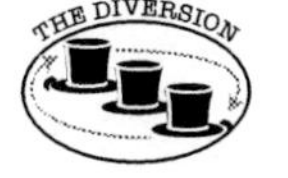


*The noting of her "scratching more than usual" is likewise there to lead you to believe that the patient has been sexually abused.*

*The fact that she fell on a chair is an incidental finding. It would not explain the findings on physical exam.*

*Bouts of constipation can be the result of abuse however it could also be the result of whatever is causing the genital and now presumed anogenital itching. It will also explain the anal fissure noted on physical examination further in the question.*

 

*(Continued from previous page)*

The parents are married and the patient has a 5-year-old brother and a 10-year-old sister. There have not been any houseguests recently and the mother takes care of the child before and after school. When the mother asked the child she denied that anyone has touched her privates.

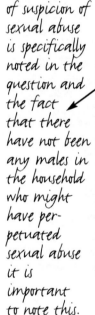

PERTINENT NEGATIVE

*When denial of suspicion of sexual abuse is specifically noted in the question and the fact that there have not been any males in the household who might have perpetuated sexual abuse it is important to note this.*

On physical examination you note that the hymen is intact with a continuous inner edge, the posterior fourchette does not appear to be friable.

*Important physical finding which points away from sexual abuse.*

However you do note that the labia majora appear to be mildly excoriated with 2 small blood blisters and some dried blood. The labia appear pale and atrophic. The anal opening is within normal limits for age with a small anal fissure, which is barely noticeable.

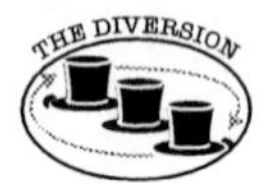


*These are classic signs for lichens sclerosis and therefore should help solidify the diagnosis.*

## Question 1:

A) Lichen Sclerosus

## Question 2:

D) High potency steroid cream

Lichen sclerosus is a dermatological condition that involves the skin of the perineum. Consistent with the vignette in this question the hymen and mucosal tissue are not involved and are normal on physical exam.

However skin involving the anus and outer vaginal tissue including the vulva can become *hypopigmented* and *atrophic*. The lesions are quite pruritic and therefore the patients tend to scratch a lot. This leads to the blood blisters, excoriation and dried blood seen in this patient.

In addition the anus can be involved leading to painful defecation, which is what leads to constipation. The constipation can result in the anal fissure seen in this patient, which can easily be mistaken for further substantiation of sexual abuse.

Sexual abuse can occur with no physical findings. However, when they do present with physical findings one would expect to see signs of trauma including breaching the integrity of the hymen as well of signs of trauma in the vestibule. Vaginal foreign body would more likely present with foul odor and discharge. Likewise physiologic vaginitis would present with discharge as an important presenting feature.

PERIL WARNING It is important to note that sexual abuse can occur even in a patient who happens to have Lichen Sclerosus. It wouldn't be prudent to read too much into a question like this since the correct answer will likely be Lichen Sclerosus. However, if you had an unclear history with concern for sexual abuse and if you are given two choices for management:

A) High potency steroids
*and*
B) Sexual abuse
C) Sexual abuse evaluation

The correct answer will be B since you must be sure sexual abuse did not occur.

# Case 5

(see page 17 for Questions)

A 14-year-old girl presents with a one-week history of vague symptoms of malaise, nausea and poor appetitive. Her last menstrual period was a week ago and she had a low-grade fever, which has since resolved.

On physical exam you note several small edematous papules on the hands and face.

This is a description of Gianotti-Crosti syndrome

Her serum IgM/IgG EBV titers were negative; her Serum beta HCG is negative. Her liver function tests are markedly elevated and her CBC is within normal limits.

You suspect acute Hepatitis B infection.

This is one of those questions where they give you a whole song and dance and then give you the diagnosis.

 

## Question 1:

C) Anti- HBs

## Question 2:

A) Anti –HBc

## Question 3:

A) HBsAg and Anti-Hbe

The following table will enable you to answer this and any question regarding the convoluted serology of Hepatitis B:

| Alphabet Convolution Measured | What the heck it is! | What it means (if positive) for you on the exam! |
|---|---|---|
| Anti-HBs | Antibody to Surface Antigen | Immunity due to viral infection that was cleared **or** to immunization |
| HbsAg | Surface antigen | Acute infection, Late Incubation period, Healthy carrier, or Chronic infection |
| HbeAg | e- antigen | Active replication of the virus and, of course, this person is very infective- stay away if you can!<br>Can occur during :<br>1. acute infection,<br>2. late incubation,<br>3. chronic infection. |

| | | |
|---|---|---|
| Anti Hbe | Antibody to e-antigen | Anti Hbe is<br>· positive in healthy carriers<br>· negative in chronic disease<br>INSIDER TIPS Healthy carrier as indicated by the concurrent presence of HbsAg, they will have a low level of infectivity and are safe |
| IgM Anti-HBc | IgM Antibody to Core Antigen | This is an IgM antibody - therefore it arrives early and leaves early and is therefore a reflection of acute disease.<br>PERIL WARNING Can also be positive in healthy carriers and chronic disease, just to make it really confusing. |
| Anti-HBc | Either IgG or IgM core antibody.<br>INSIDER TIPS If not specified, implies IgG antibody. | Would be present during acute disease and later on reflecting both past and present disease and therefore not very helpful in pinpointing timing of disease by itself.<br>INSIDER TIPS Highly positive in Chronic disease and in healthy carriers. |
| HBV DNA | Reflects Hepatitis B viremia | Indicates active replication of disease and therefore active disease |

# Case 6

(see page 19 for Questions)

You are evaluating a 12-year-old boy who was hit on the left eye by a baseball. There was no loss of consciousness and he has been alert and responsive since with no vomiting or significant headache.

Subdural and epidural hematoma ruled out

The sclera is injected and he squints when the lights are turned on and he is very uncomfortable.

Photophobia

On ophthalmologic exam you do not see any blood in the anterior chamber of the eye; the eye is equal and reactive with a normal funduscopic examination. Vision screen shows a slight decreased visual acuity in the impacted eye but he can see.

PERTINENT NEGATIVE

Hyphema ruled out

Detached retina ruled out

## Question 1:

C) Traumatic iritis

## Question 2:

E) Slit lamp eye exam

## Question 3:

C) Ketorolac eyedrops and followup

In this patient the combination of photophobia, slight visual deficit with a normal EOM, pupillary response and funduscopic exam, the only remaining diagnosis is *traumatic iritis.* The most appropriate diagnostic step in this case would be a slit lamp exam and treatment with ketorolac eyedrops and followup.

 

# Case 7

*(see page 21 for Questions)*

You grab your chart off the rack and see on the triage note that it is an 8-year-old with abdominal pain and fever. You enter the room to find a child playing and laughing, as he tears the paper off the examining table and drapes it over his parents. You excuse yourself to find the actual room with the patient. His mother jumps up, trailing the examination table paper behind her, and tells you this is the right room.

THE DIVERSION

He is an otherwise healthy very active boy. In fact, he is being treated with methylphenidate for ADHD but only during the week. The family has several pets and the boy plays with them all weekend.

Pure Diversion

Whenever they note pets it is never irrelevant

*(Continued on next page)*

*(Continued from previous page)*

Although the boy looks great now, mom says you should see him around midnight when he is doubled over in pain lasting several hours. The next day he is fit as a fiddle. He has had no vomiting or diarrhea.

Summarized as, episodic abdominal pain and fever spikes

This should tell you that Chrons disease is very unlikely since growth retardation would be part of the picture

On Physical examination the boy is tall for his age, vigorous and in better shape than you.

He is afebrile with vital signs stable. There is no rash noted, just several linear scabs on the arm the parents attribute to his horsing around with the pets.

Linear scabs or scratches and the word pet in the same sentence should alert you to the possibility of Cat Scratch Disease

Abdomen- soft, non-tender, with no guarding or rebound tenderness.

You admit the patient and, sure enough, confirm the spiking temperature and the acute episodic abdominal pain.

Whatever is going on it is real since it is confirmed by the hospital staff

 

## Question 1:

D) Microabscesses of the liver

## Question 2:

D) *Bartonella henselae*

## Question 3:

C) Azithromycin

Indeed this is a very atypical presentation of cat scratch disease and when hepatic microabscesses develop, intermittent acute abdominal pain and fever spikes would be a typical presentation of this atypical development; but prime real estate for the board exam. *Bartonella henselae* would be the etiologic agent and of all the choices in question 3 Azithromycin would be the best choice.

# Case 8

(see page 25 for Questions)

Eye pain precedes swelling

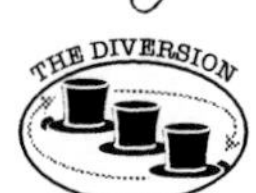


Rubbing eye is a diversion and not relevant

A 15-year-old boy presents with a one-week history of cough and upper respiratory infection symptoms. His right eye has been bothering him and has hurt each time he rubs it, which he admits is a lot of time since he cannot resist the temptation. He presents today because he developed a fever and the right eyelid and surrounding tissue is now red and swollen. All of his immunizations are up to date.

Presentation preceded by URI and cough

Periorbital erythema and swelling

Makes H. Flu type b unlikely

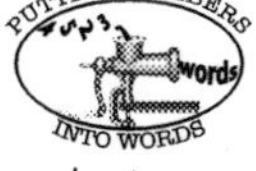


Febrile

Physical exam confirms a temperature of 101.3 F with marked periorbital swelling, periorbital tenderness and proptosis. His extraocular movements appear to be intact with the exception of upward gaze, which he has difficulty with.

Decreased EOM

## Question 1:

B) Orbital cellulitis

## Question 2:

C) *S. pyogenes*

You being presented with a patient who

- Initially had a URI
- Has Eye Pain
- Developed into periorbital swelling, erythema, pain with decreased EOMI who is febrile

This all points to *orbital cellulitis*, which is typically caused by: *Staph aureus* (common in neonates and children older than 5), *Strep Pyogenes* (common in children older than 5), *Strep pneumoniae* (most common in age 6 months to 5 years and one of the most common in children older than 5) and *H. Influenza.*

In this case, *H. Influenza* is unlikely since the child received all immunizations. In addition, the choices included *H. Influenza* non-typeable, which would not cause orbital cellulitis.

PERIL WARNING *Staph epidermidis* is quite a diversion since you are told that the patient rubbed his eye a lot leading you to believe that this could be the cause.

Among the choices listed as the possible etiological agent the most likely cause would be *S. pyogenes.*

# Case 9

(see page 27 for Questions)

At first glance sounds like a routine viral illness

A 7-year-old girl presents with a 7-day history of fever and vomiting. She tells you that she is feeling miserable and has no energy. 4 days ago she developed a rash on her hands and feet which is also present on her back and belly. At that time the family was visiting relatives out of town and the patient was seen in the local emergency room where they got "blood tests" and gave her an IV and some medicines.

This is a hint at the correct diagnosis of Rocky Mountain Spotted Fever

You call the ER and confirm that she received IV fluids for dehydration and was given IV Ceftriaxone. Blood cultures are negative.

A hint at a bacterial etiology as a diversion

On physical exam she is ill-appearing with a rash on her trunk, abdomen, feet and hands which can be best described

(Continued on next page)

*(Continued from previous page)*

as maculopapular and blanching.

You also note some scattered petechiae on her hands and ankles.

Classic RMSF description. This should help you nail the diagnosis

Temperature-101.6
HR-130
RR- 45
BP – 80/40

PUTTING NUMBERS INTO WORDS

Febrile, Tachycardia, Hypotension

HEENT- dry mucous membranes, EOMI, PERRLA. TM intact, non-injected. Throat – clear
Neck – Supple

Card – S1S2 no murmur
Abdomen – Soft, non-tender, no guarding, decreased bowel sounds.

Abdominal symptoms are consistent with a diagnosis of RMSF

*(Continued on next page)*

*(Continued from previous page)*

LABS:

CBC- H/H 9/27

WBC- 4.5 82 neutrophils 15

Lymphocytes 3 Monos

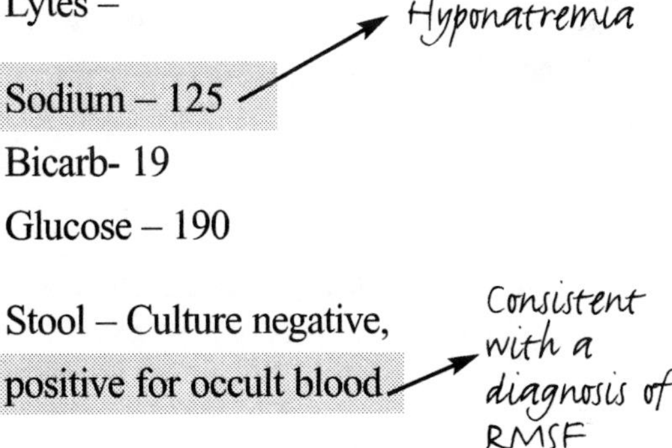

Lytes –
Sodium – 125
Hyponatremia
Bicarb- 19
Glucose – 190
Stool – Culture negative,
positive for occult blood
Consistent with a diagnosis of RMSF

## Question 1:

E) Indirect fluorescent antibody testing 7-10 days after the onset of illness

## Question 2:

C) Rocky Mountain Spotted Fever

## Question 3:

A) Doxycycline IV or PO

The child in this vignette is presenting with classic signs and symptoms of Rocky Mountain Spotted Fever (RMSF). Classic presenting signs include general signs such as fever, headache, nausea, vomiting, diarrhea and malaise. More specific signs include *abdominal pain* and a rash that start starts out as maculopapular, which later becomes petechial, concentrated on the feet and hands.

*The absence of rash does not rule out RMSF*, since it is absent 20% of the time, however on the boards they are almost obligated to describe this pattern to distinguish it from other illnesses in the differential.

Most cases occur during the warm months between April and September, typically in the Southeastern and South Central United States.

INSIDER TIPS Long Island is another location where one can contract RMSF, which is often a diversion on board exams.

The typical **lab findings of RMSF** include *hyponatremia* and *thrombocytopenia* as seen in this patient.

 

PERIL WARNING The definitive diagnosis is by documented antibodies to R. rickettsii *7-10 days after the onset of symptoms*. This will often be negative at the onset of illness and does not rule out RMSF. Therefore waiting for definitive diagnosis is never correct. If you are presented with a patient with symptoms suggestive of RMSF who has traveled to a region endemic for RMSF then immediate treatment is the correct answer.

In addition LFTs can sometimes be elevated which was not noted in this vignette.

Ceftriaxone would be ineffective in **treating RMSF** thus the clinical deterioration of this patient despite treatment with IV ceftriaxone. The best treatment is Doxycycline.

INSIDER TIPS This is one instance where doxycycline would be the correct treatment even in children younger than 8. The risk of staining teeth is minimal during one course of doxycycline and certainly the morbidity of untreated RMSF outweighs the risk of stained teeth.

# Case 10

(see page 31 for Questions)

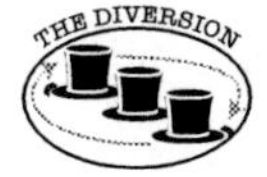


You are asked to evaluate a 10-year-old boy who is currently at the 95th%ile for weight and 5th percentile for height. Up until age 7 the child was at the 75th% ile for both weight and height. He is currently taking no medication and his appetite has not changed-his diet is nutritionally balanced. On physical exam, in addition to marked obesity, you notice several small bruises on his hands and feet.

*short and obese*

*simultaneous increase in weight and decrease in height, consistent with an* ***endocrine disorder***

PERTINENT NEGATIVE

*No exogenous medications as a cause*

PERTINENT NEGATIVE

*Points away from diagnosis of Prader Willi*

*Easy bruisability*

(Continued on next page)

(Continued from previous page)

LABS

Leukocytosis with no left shift

CBC

WBC- 19.5

45% neutrophils 45% lymphocytes

10% monocytes

Hypokalemia

Na/ 139 K/ 2.5 Cl/105 Bicarb/ 25

Glucose/ 75 Bun/ 19 Cre/ 0.4

## Question 1:

D) Cushing Syndrome

## Question 2:

D) Dexamethasone suppression study

In this patient we have a simultaneous decrease in height and increase in weight on the growth curve. This is consistent with an endocrine disorder, either Cushing syndrome or hypothyroid.

Children with Prader Willi syndrome will be short but will also have a history of hyperphagia or as it are known in the real world, "eating a lot". The decrease in height on the growth curve is also inconsistent with a diagnosis of Prader Willi syndrome

The easy bruisability, leukocytosis, hypokalemia suggests a diagnosis of Cushing syndrome. This diagnosis is best confirmed with the Dexamethasone suppression study.

# Case 11

*(see page 35 for Questions)*

You are called to the nursery to evaluate a full term female baby that according to the nurse "may have ambiguous genitalia". The baby has been feeding well and has been in no distress, except for some difficulty breast-feeding, which is being managed by the lactation counselor. The prenatal course has been unremarkable and the mother denies taking any medication. She was negative for group B strep.

*Anything in quotes is not an established fact*

THE DIVERSION

*Red herring normal finding*

*Anything denied is not an established fact*

On physical exam the infant is well hydrated, good skin turgor and cap refill < 2 seconds.

*No signs of salt wasting or shock*

*(Continued on next page)*

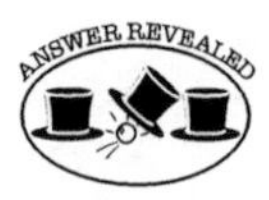


Virilization but not ambiguous genitalia

*(Continued from previous page)*

Examination of the external genitalia reveals a symmetrical swelling of the labia majora, and definite rugae and slight increased pigmentation. There is no clitoromegaly with a normal vaginal and urethral opening. Good urine output is demonstrated with the baby urinating on the blanket you just placed in the bassinet.

LABS

Na/ 139 K/ 4.9 Cl/ 109 Bun/ 14
Cre/ 0.3 Glucose/ 97
CBC- WBC 5.6, normal differential
Platelets – 210 K
H/H 14/45

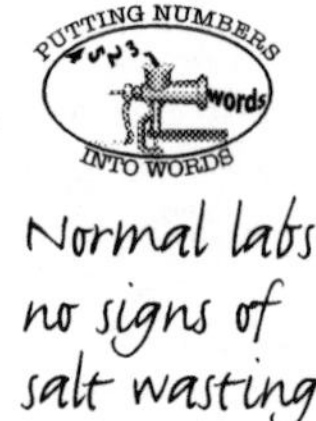


Normal labs no signs of salt wasting

 

## Question 1:

E) Reassurance of nurse and parents in that order

## Question 2:

E) Exogenous androgens

In this case the documentation of the urethral opening and the vaginal opening rules out ambiguous genitalia. However the hyperpigmentation and the rugae are indicative of virilization and the only explanation could be exogenous androgens despite mother's denial. Therefore the only intervention would be reassurance.

You would also know that congenital adrenal hyperplasia is not the diagnosis by the normal lab findings and the overall well being of the infant.

 

# Case 12

(see page 39 for Questions)

A 2-year-old presents with a one day history of profuse watery diarrhea, occasionally green in color with no blood noted. Last night he vomited twice and had a tactile temperature with mild abdominal pain. He has not been taking in any PO fluids and it is not clear if he has had any urine output since his stool is too watery.

*Profuse watery diarrhea with low-grade fever and vomiting and mild abdominal pain suggests a viral gastroenteritis.*

The parents deny any exposure to toxic substances, and, except for a course of amoxicillin a month ago, he is taking no other medications and he has not eaten any spoiled food. There are 3 children from his daycare who also have diarrhea. His past medical history is unremarkable.

*No exposure to toxic substances or to spoiled foods points away from an etiology of food poisoning*

(Continued on next page)

*(Continued from previous page)*

On physical exam you note the child to be listless with dry mucous membranes.
Afebrile, HR 150, RR 25, BP 85/60
Cap refill > 3 seconds with extremities cool to touch.
HEENT- TMs intact, no erythema
Mouth – Dry mucous membranes
Throat – Clear, no erythema or exudate
Lungs – Clear
Card – S1S2 No murmur
Neuro – Lethargic, symmetric tone, with DTR 2+ throughout

PUTTING NUMBERS INTO WORDS

Tachycardia with increased cap refill

These factors point out that the patient is markedly dehydrated and would need IV fluid hydration to restore electrolyte balance. IV fluids overnight would be preferred over PO hydration.

LAB FINDINGS:

CBC

WBC 11.5
Hgb 12 HCT 36.5 Segs 55%

*(Continued on next page)*

 

*(Continued from previous page)*

Lymphs 40%   Monocytes 5%
Platelets 220

Lytes
Sodium 136   Potassium 4.5
Bicarb 14   BUN 32   Cre 0.5

UA (cath)

Sp Gravity 1.050   pH 5.2
Glucose negative   Ketones Large
WBC- 2   RBC – 2
Bacteria – negative

These factors point out that the patient is markedly dehydrated and would need IV fluid hydration to restore electrolyte balance. IV fluids overnight would be preferred over PO hydration.

 

## Question 1:

C) Rotavirus antigen testing

## Question 2:

D) IV hydration and overnight admission

## Question 3:

D) Hand washing

The correct answer for Question 1 is Choice C since the most likely etiology is viral, specifically rotavirus. Since the patient is afebrile, bacterial causes such as Salmonella are unlikely. Therefore the correct treatment would be IV hydration and overnight admission due to the delayed cap refill and low serum bicarb.

The most effective way to prevent rotavirus is through hand washing. All of the other choices do not apply here. (However, a rotavirus vaccine is in the pipeline – no pun intended.)

PERIL WARNING **C. Diff diarrhea is rarely associated with severe dehydration.**

 

# Case 13

(see page 43 for Questions)

A 21month-old toddler was found by his mother vomiting, coughing and gagging. The mother had just returned from shopping and the child was with his 17 year-old baby-sitter who noted that the toddler did go into the garage 20 minutes earlier for not more than 5 minutes while she ran to the kitchen to turn off the stove, which had been on for quite a while.

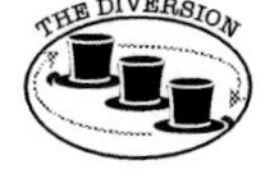


This is a distracter attempting to make you believe that carbon monoxide poisoning is the diagnosis.

Vomiting, coughing, gagging possibly due to exposure to a chemical substance

The child has no past medical history of any respiratory problems including asthma. There are no household members or recent visitors who are taking any prescription medications.

This points away from a diagnosis of asthma or pneumonia.

The toddler is brought to see you in the pediatric ER because the toddler cannot stop coughing and gagging.

*(Continued on next page)*

*(Continued from previous page)*

On physical exam the child is afebrile with a HR 125, BP 90/50, $SaO_2$ 92% on room air. RR 45, Lungs are clear to auscultation, no wheeze or rales. He is tachypneic and coughing.

PERTINENT NEGATIVE

This points away from a diagnosis of asthma or pneumonia.

Tachypnea

## Question 1:

D) Hydrocarbon ingestion

## Question 2:

D) Give supplemental $O_2$

## Question 3:

C) CXR and observation with repeat CXR in 6 hours

This history and findings in this vignette would be consistent with a patient who has a hydrocarbon ingestion or aspiration such as kerosene. This could easily occur in the "5 minutes" the child spent in the garage unsupervised.

In addition to tachypnea, the child is hypoxic. Therefore, before any diagnostic studies are done it is important to stick to the ABCs and therefore administration of oxygen comes before x-ray. CXR would be appropriate but it would not be the most appropriate *next step.*

Since one of the mainstays of treatment is the prevention of emesis syrup of ipecac would not only be the wrong choice; it is contraindicated.

Once oxygen is given then a CXR would be appropriate. However with hydrocarbon ingestion and/or aspiration the initial CXR will likely be negative. Therefore it needs to be repeated in 4-6 hours.

If the repeat CXR is negative → the parents should be given detailed instructions on the early signs of respiratory compromise and should be seen in followup within 24 hours. This is because pneumonitis can develop within 12-24 hours.

 

If the repeat CXR is positive → the child should of course be admitted.

If carbon monoxide poisoning would be the correct diagnosis high oxygen saturation would be part of the presentation, not a low one. In addition, this is not the clinical presentation you would expect with carbon monoxide poisoning. Carbon monoxide poisoning would typically present with lethargy.

---

Ref: Fleisher, Ludwig. *Textbook of Pediatric Emergency Medicine.* 2000; pg. 912- 914

# Case 14

(see page 47 for Questions)

An 18-year-old girl presents with a 3-day history of abdominal pain and vomiting, which is worsening. She is afebrile and has had no diarrhea.

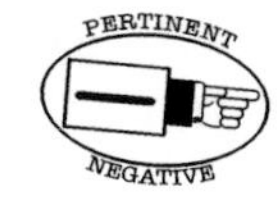


No diarrhea points away from a viral gastroenteritis

She has had intermittent abdominal pain over the past 6 months diagnosed as irritable bowel syndrome. She is non-icteric. The pain is dull at the moment but can be sharp and she sometimes experiences back pain as well.

Incorrectly diagnosed as irritable bowel syndrome

Radiating to the back suggests pancreatitis

THE DIVERSION

Denies alcohol use

While alcohol abuse is associated with pancreatitis in adults this association is not as strong in pancreatitis in children

She is not sexually active and is not taking birth control pills. Denies drinking alcohol or any illicit drug use.

Past history is significant for a diagnosis of bipolar depression at age 15 for which she is being treated

(Continued on next page)

Noting Valproic acid is not incidental. They are telling you that a side effect of Valproic Acid could be the cause of the abdominal pain.

*(Continued from previous page)*

with valproic acid as a mood stabilizer. Her levels were last checked 10 days ago and were within therapeutic range.

On physical examination she is non-icteric. Her vital signs are stable. On abdominal exam her pain is mostly epigastric and left upper quadrant with no guarding or rebound tenderness. There is no hepatosplenomegaly and bowel sounds are normal.

Important physical findings to identify the source of the pain

Her mouth is dry and the remainder of the exam is unremarkable.

Dry mouth just tells you she is dehydrated and too non-specific to help with the question

LABORATORY FINDINGS

WBC – 14.5 H/H 15/45

Platelets – 238 K

*(Continued on next page)*

*(Continued from previous page)*

Sodium/ 140 Potassium/ 4.0

Chloride/ 105 Bicarb/22

Glucose/ 145 Bun/9

Creatinine/0.2

Aspartate aminotransferase/189

Alanine aminotransferase/338

Alkaline phosphatase/324

Elevated LFT's and other labs suggesting obstructive jaundice

Bilirubin-

Total 2.5 Direct/ 1.4

PUTTING NUMBERS INTO WORDS

Hyper-bilirubinemia

Total Protein/7.4 Albumin/4.2

Calcium/9.2

ABG 7.45/36/68

Oxygen Saturation – 98 % on Room Air

Abdominal Ultrasound – multiple gallstones and no focal pancreatic lesions

## Question 1:

A) Serum Amylase and Lipase

## Question 2:

B) Meperidine

## Question 3:

D) Hypoglycemia

The patient in the vignette has a diagnosis of acute gallstone pancreatitis. Additional contributing factors would be valproic acid, which is also associated with acute pancreatitis.

THE DIVERSION By mentioning that the patient is taking valproic acid for a mood disorder they are diverting you into believing that irritable bowel syndrome which is also associated with emotional problems is behind the problem, but this is just a trick since the pain is too severe and longstanding to be passed off as irritable bowel syndrome.

It is also important to note that although pancreatitis presents as epigastric pain that sometimes radiates to the right side it can also present as left sided upper quadrant tenderness, as is the case in this vignette.

Since they already note that there are gallstones in the gallbladder and confirm the presence of obstructive hyperbilirubinemia the best way to confirm the diagnosis at this point is by obtaining a serum amylase and lipase.

Elevated serum lipase is associated with acute pancreatitis. Acute pancreatitis can be caused by hypercalcemia, but it can also lead to hypocalcemia as a metabolic complication. *Therefore both hypercalcemia and hypocalcemia are associated with acute pancreatitis.* Because of decreased insulin levels hyperglycemia is associated with pancreatitis and hypoglycemia is not.

Regarding the immediate treatment of gallstone pancreatitis-Endoscopic retrograde cholangiopancreatography or ERCP as it is more commonly known in the street and in the hospital may not be indicated right away since gallstones can actually pass spontaneously in children.

Since morphine can cause spasm and worsen pancreatitis, meperidine is the preferred pain management in patients with acute pancreatitis.

# Case 15

(see page 51 for Questions)

A 14-year-old boy is brought in by EMS after being discovered in the garage by his parents obtunded after one episode of emesis. His mother reported that he had complained earlier of blurred vision.

His father had been in the garage the previous night winterizing the car and doing other work on the engine. Several chemicals were left in one-liter soda bottles on the work bench, as noted by the paramedics on the scene. The patient also enjoys working on cars and has frequently worked with his dad. He is also an honor student.

Antifreeze ingestion likely

On Physical examination:
No odor of alcohol was noted on the breath and has had no history of drinking alcohol.

*(Continued on next page)*

*(Continued from previous page)*

PUTTING NUMBERS INTO WORDS

Vital Signs:
Afebrile, Respiratory Rate – 36 per minute, HR – 160, and BP 140/85

Tachypnea, Tachycardia, mild hypertension

The lungs were clear. Cardiac – 2+ pulses, cap refill < 2 seconds, normal sinus rhythm with no murmurs. Abdominal exam – soft, non-tender, no guarding or rebound tenderness. No organomegaly. Neurological exam- The patient appears to be lethargic and groggy. 2+ DTR throughout with symmetrical tone and strength.

PUTTING NUMBERS INTO WORDS

The anion gap is 146 – (107 + 14) = 25

Therefore you need to write in the margin, "Elevated anion gap"

LABORATORY FINDINGS –
Sodium 146 mEq/L,
Potassium 4.2 mEq/L,
Chloride 107 mEq/L,
Bicarbonate 14 mEq/L,
Serum urea nitrogen 12 mg/dL,

*(Continued on next page)*

*(Continued from previous page)*

Creatinine 0.9 mg/dL,

Blood glucose 148 mg/dL,

Total serum calcium 10 mg/dL,

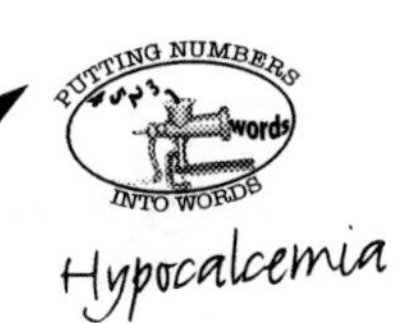


Phosphorus 5.1 mg/dL,

Magnesium 2.8 mg/dL.

Urinalysis was normal, with the exception of the presence of calcium oxalate crystals.

Arterial blood gas:

pH 7.12,

PaO2 71 mm Hg,

PCO2 30 mm Hg.

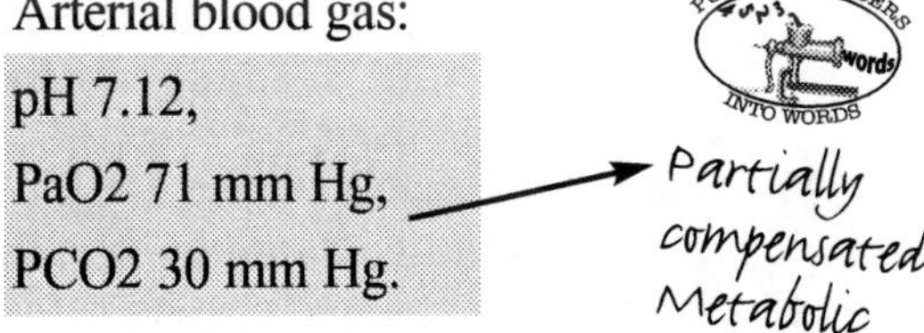


 

## Question 1:

B) Ethylene glycol

## Question 2:

E) Intubation

## Question 3:

C) Renal Failure

The clinical vignette depicts a patient who most likely ingested ethylene glycol, which, given its sweet taste can easily be mistakenly ingested, especially if inappropriately stored in a soda bottle.

Metabolic acidosis, hypocalcemia as well as tachycardia, hypertension and tachypnea are all signs of ethylene glycol ingestion. The presence of oxalate crystals in the urine should be a dead giveaway.

In any patient who is obtunded, especially one with metabolic acidosis, the first step to take is intubation to protect the airway until the patient is stabilized. The long term complications of ethylene glycol ingestion, especially if not taken care of immediately include renal failure. However, early recognition and intervention should reduce this risk significantly.

Ref: Fleisher, Ludwig. *Textbook of Pediatric Emergency Medicine.* 2000; 903-904.

 

# Case 16

(see page 55 for Questions)

You are asked to see a 22-month-old girl because of developmental delay and odd features that your family practice colleague cannot quite identify. The child's physical growth was on target for the first year but then trailed off. The girl is not walking yet and has not spoken any complete words.

Cannot be an X-linked recessive disorder

Normal physical growth first year, developmental delay

The child has had an extraordinary number of respiratory infections. You agree that the child does have some odd features including a rather large head and a face that is a bit too harsh, especially for a female; as well as an enlarged tongue and corneal clouding. Exam is also significant for hepatomegaly and a 3/6 systolic ejection murmur.

Chronic respiratory infections that are clinically significant

Coarse facies, enlarged tongue, corneal clouding and macrocephaly.

Hepatomegaly and cardiac insufficiency

 

## Question 1:

D) Measure urine mucopolysaccharide (GAG) levels

## Question 2:

D) Hurlers syndrome

## Question 3:

A) Hearing loss

The course facies should have tipped you off that this is a mucopolysaccharidoses and therefore the correct study would be to measure urine mucopolysaccharide levels.

Urine mucopolysaccharide levels would be the correct answer here because here because they asked for the best *initial* step to take.

However if they asked for the most *definitive test* step it would be serum *enzymes* since this is more definitive.

This should also limit you down to two choices for the correct diagnosis.

It is very important when reading a question that involves a female that you write in the margins "cannot be x-linked recessive". In this case once you have narrowed this down to a mucopolysaccharidoses, you would be down to two choices, Hurlers and Hunters-and if you had done your homework and knew that Hunters was x-linked you could cross this choice out without batting an eyelash. Hunters can present with and without mental impairment and developmental delay.[1] However corneal clouding is not seen in Hunters syndrome.

This leaves you with the only possible correct choice, Hurler's syndrome, which is associated with chronic respiratory infections and cardiac insufficiency, which was suggested on the physical findings. Additional findings can include hearing loss and increased *intracranial pressure*

[1] See *Laughing Your Way to Passing the Pediatric Boards ® 3rd edition* for a simple mnemonic on this and other diseases and their inheritance patterns/associated features; for example, you shouldn't hunt if you have corneal clouding.

 

# Case 17

*(see page 57 for Questions)*

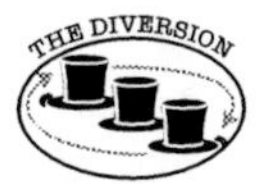


Bad cough and chest tightness could be consistent with reactive airway disease/asthma or pneumonia, which would be the first thing that comes to mind in both cases

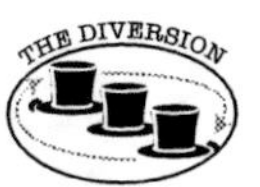


You are evaluating a 16-year-old girl who for the past week has had a "bad cold and cough". The cold has gotten "a little better" but the cough has remained the same and her chest also feels tight and her chest hurts. The pain is intermittent but seems to get worse when she lies down. In addition, she has experienced RUQ tenderness, back pain and some nausea and vomiting.

RUQ tenderness would divert you toward a diagnosis of gall bladder or liver disease.

Vomiting, back pain and even RUQ tenderness would divert you toward a diagnosis of pyelonephritis or kidney stones.

Her past medical history is unremarkable and other than oral contraceptive pills she is not taking and has never been prescribed any medications.

THE DIVERSION

Using language like "other than" automatically leads you believe this medication is not important, unless you make that extra step to note this could simply be an attempt to divert you from its importance.

*(Continued on next page)*

*(Continued from previous page)*

**Physical Exam:**

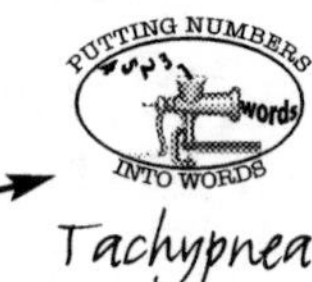


Temp – 99.1
Respiratory Rate- 25 → Tachypnea
HR- 101

She is in no apparent distress at rest
HEENT – throat clear, TMs intact, non-injected
Neck – supple, no palpable lymph nodes
Lungs – Clear, no wheeze, rales or rhonchi
Card – S1 S2, normal sinus rhythm, 2+ pulses throughout with cap refill < 2 seconds
Abdomen- soft, mild RUQ tenderness with no guarding or rebound, no hepatosplenomegaly
Back – mild right-sided flank pain.

THE DIVERSION

These can be consistent with other diagnoses but as pointed out below it is also consistent with a diagnosis of pulmonary embolus

*(Continued on next page)*

 

(Continued from previous page)

**Laboratory studies –**

Venous Doppler ultrasound / Legs – Negative

This is the mother of all diversions. The negative Doppler does not rule out pulmonary embolus

 

## Question 1:

D) Chest CT

## Question 2:

D) Pulmonary embolus

## Question 3:

E) Heparin and Warfarin

The classic presentation of a pulmonary embolus is:

1) Pleuritic chest pain
2) Dyspnea
3) Hemoptysis

However, other less specific and often misleading signs and symptoms can also be a part of the picture including *back pain* and *mild abdominal pain.* In up to one-half of cases the Doppler ultrasound of the legs can be negative, especially if the source of the embolus is in the pelvic veins or elsewhere.

It would be important to note the importance of the oral contraceptive pills since this is a key part of the history, despite the downplaying of its importance in the wording of the question.

If you were to be presented with other diagnostic options other than CT scan of the chest here are some important points to consider:

- **Ventilation / Perfusion Scan** – If it is negative, it rules out embolism. However, in a non-high probability scan, positive results are not conclusive. Therefore, it would not be the correct choice if other more specific studies were available.

 

- **Pulmonary angiography** – This is very accurate, however with a 5% morbidity rate and high expense, it is rarely used and would not likely be the correct answer.
- **Spiral CT of the Chest** – This would be the more appropriate study, especially in a low-probability case.
- **D-dimers** – 80 % of patients with venous thromboemboli will have a positive result. Therefore, this could be a correct answer if it is included among the choices, especially as evidence in conjunction with CT.

The proper treatment would be low molecular weight heparin and warfarin.

# Case 18

(see page 61 for Questions)

You are evaluating a 12-year-old girl who has just recovered from a recent viral illness and has been having difficulty walking over the past few days. You note weakness in her legs with deep tendon reflexes of 1+. Upper extremity strength is normal with deep tendon reflexes 2+. There is no point tenderness over the vertebral spine and MRI earlier this week was negative.

Ascending paralysis

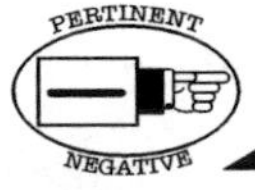


Transverse myelitis and ruptured disc unlikely

## Question 1:

C) Respiratory arrest

## Question 2:

B) Lumbar puncture

## Question 3:

E) Guillain Barré disease

The combination of ascending paralysis in the aftermath of a viral illness is most suggestive of a diagnosis of Guillain Barré disease. The respiratory failure is the most serious concern since it can come on rapidly and is often the cause of death in this setting. Of the choices given the best way to diagnose Guillain Barré disease is by lumbar puncture. If EMG were one of the choices it too would be correct.

 

# Case 19

(see page 63 for Questions)

The description of the rash is classic for neonatal lupus

You are called to the nursery at 6:30 AM just prior to change of shift to evaluate a newborn with a concerning rash. The baby was born full-term with an uneventful prenatal course and normal spontaneous vaginal delivery.

On Physical exam you note a skin eruption on the infant's face and scalp which is a violaceous-dusky color with skin atrophy in the middle of papular scaly eruptions. There is no hepatosplenomegaly on physical exam. Lungs are clear to auscultation and heart sounds are normal, S1S2 with no murmur.

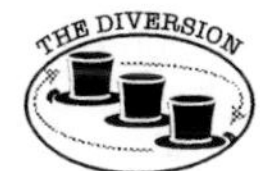


Since neonatal lupus is associated with 3rd degree heart block this is placed in the question to throw you off the trail. Only 50% of reported cases present with heart block

Mild Thrombocytopenia, also consistent with neonatal lupus.

**CBC-**

WBC- 9.5

H/H – 36/12

Platelet Count 125

EKG- Unremarkable

## Question 1:

E) Serum anti-Ro (ssA) level

## Question 2:

D) Discharge and judicious use of sun block

## Question 3:

E) Ganciclovir and Foscarnet

The answer to Question 1 would be Serum anti-Rho (sSA) level. If maternal were one of the choices this too would have been correct since the described rash is consistent with neonatal lupus. All of the associated signs of neonatal lupus are due to the transplacental transfer of the anti-Rho antibodies which is a short lived problem.

The correct answer to Question 2 is choice D.

Typically the described rash does not appear until several weeks or months since it is the binding of these antibodies to skin which is potentiated by the exposure to ultraviolet light.

Therefore if you actually lost points for picking an absolutely wrong answer then you would lose extra points for picking choice E, exposure to indirect light. This is would make this rash worse. The rash is not altogether benign. It can lead telangiectasias, scarring and atrophy needing laser therapy. Therefore it is important to use sun block until the antibodies are out of the system several months later.

While the rash typically presents several months later after exposure to sunlight it can indeed present in the immediate newborn period as it did in the patient in this case study.

 

Question 3 is a bit unfair since CMV is not the correct diagnosis. But who said the board exam is fair. You know what they say, all is fair in love and boards.

Besides you didn't expect us to give you the answer with one of the questions. The only time this would happen on the boards is when you cannot go back to the previous question either on the electronic format of the pediatric recertification exam or a book given on a previous day on the certification exam.

The answer is choice E Ganciclovir and Foscarnet. Both are approved for the treatment of CMV retinitis. Ganciclovir is the first line treatment and foscarnet is reserved for when ganciclovir fails. Amantadine is indicated to treat influenza A. Acyclovir and Vidarabine are used to treat HSV infection and varicella. Ribavirin is reserved for RSV virus in specific instances. Zapemall is one we made up for comic relief, as in "Zap them all".

 

# Case 20

(see page 65 for Questions)

A 6-year-old with a one-week history of vomiting presents to your office.

THE DIVERSION

Consistent with viral GE which is not the correct diagnosis

He is afebrile, with no diarrhea. He was seen in the emergency room last night while the parents were driving home from a camping trip. He was prescribed promethazine suppositories and told to followup with you. He has had no episodes of vomiting last night and has remained afebrile.

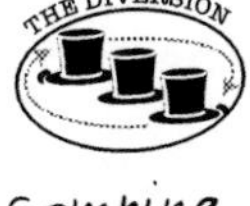


Camping trip to divert you into believing this is due to Giardia Lamblia

The parents are concerned because he appears to be weak and he is unsteady and needs some assistance standing up. He also claims that you have two heads and only one is talking.

These symptoms would be consistent with a CNS abnormality

On physical examination the child exhibits unsteady gait with diplopia.

*(Continued on next page)*

 

*(Continued from previous page)*

Other than that his neurological examination is normal with symmetrical tone and strength and 2+ DTR throughout. His abdomen is soft with no guarding, rebound or tenderness. There is no hepatosplenomegaly. He is pale with dry mucous membranes.

Non-specific findings consistent with vomiting

## Question 1:

E ) Head CT

## Question 2:

E) Arterio-venous malformation

In this question you have a patient with a set of non-specific findings including vomiting and dehydration. However, as you go through the question systematically you begin to realize that the problem most likely stems from the central nervous system.

INSIDER TIPS The combination of ataxia and vomiting suggests increased intracranial pressure

Therefore this should be a relatively easy pair of questions since only one choice in each questions focuses on the CNS.

If you were given the choice between an MRI and a head CT then the MRI would be the correct answer since MRIs are better at detecting structural abnormalities or determining the time when a hemorrhage started.

The typical presentation of an AV malformation is seizures or sequelae of hemorrhaging. Headache and focal deficits can also be part of the presenting symptoms.

 

# Case 21

(see page 69 for Questions)

A 3-month-old presents with diarrhea and is irritable with poor feeding. There is no reported history of vomiting. The stools have large "curds" in them and are yellow-brown in color.

The mother is feeding the baby modified formula in powdered form.

The child has been very irritable and mom was told by a neighbor that the child is probably hungry and she needs to make the formula stronger, which the mother says she has done.

Could be following the advice of the neighbor and concentrating the formula

PHYSICAL EXAM –

Lethargic, ill appearing
Temperature 101.2 F
HR-180
RR- 70
Weight 5 Kg

PUTTING NUMBERS INTO WORDS

Febrile, tachycardia, and tachypnea

(Continued on next page)

*(Continued from previous page)*

Skin – pale, mottled with dry mucous membranes. → Dehydration

Lungs - clear

Card – normal with weak distal pulses

Abdomen- distended, no mass, no guarding

Neuro – hyperactive, deep tendon reflexes

Skin – doughy, and redundant abdominal skin is noted.

LABS

H/H 11/33

WBC 21 with a normal differential

Sodium- 169

Potassium – 4.9

Bicarb – 15

→ Hypernatremia, Mild acidosis consistent with dehydration

*(Continued on next page)*

*(Continued from previous page)*

Bun – 25

Cre- 0.6

Urinalysis unremarkable

You diagnose hypernatremic dehydration due to increased solute loss secondary to concentrated formula.

*This is one of those cases that you read and read, and just as you are about to dislocate your shoulder congratulating yourself on making the diagnosis they come right out and tell you the diagnosis.*

## Question 1:

A) Clinical signs may be masked due to fluid shifts from intracellular to extracellular space

## Question 2:

F) Hypernatremic dehydration can result in subarachnoid and subdural hemorrhaging

In this case you have a child with hypernatremic dehydration probably secondary to a combination of fluid loss from diarrhea but more importantly from increased intake from concentrated formula. This is why you are told that the neighbor suggested this and the mother probably followed up with the advice.

The laboratory findings help establish the diagnosis that you are told in the end. The truth is these questions end up being a lot of space and time for nothing-they might as just come out and ask you a couple of questions on hypernatremic dehydration. However life and the boards aren't always that simple.

Because fluid will often shift from the intracellular space to the extracellular space, the clinical presentation is often less severe than the degree of dehydration. The sensorium often remains intact. The brain cells in response generate idiogenic osmoles, which help keep intracellular fluid from going extracellular. Unfortunately, these idiogenic osmoles stick around longer than they should and if hypernatremia is reversed too quickly you will find the cells filling up with more fluid than is needed, leading to cerebral edema and swelling. This is why hypernatremia should be corrected over 48 hours, not the 18 or 24 offered in the question.

However, if *uncorrected*, hypernatremic dehydration can result in subarachnoid and subdural hemorrhaging.

 

# Case 22

(see page 73 for Questions)

You are evaluating a 12-year-old boy with a known history of asthma. Today he received several treatments with aerosolized albuterol and continues to wheeze. On physical examination he is afebrile and has diffuse wheezing on expiration. The chest x-ray reveals some consolidation with significant volume loss on the left side.

Acute exacerbation of asthma

Afebrile, pneumonia unlikely

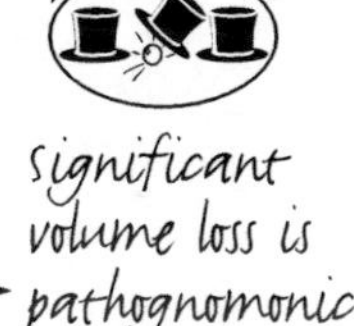


significant volume loss is pathognomonic for atelectasis

## Question 1:

A) Atelectasis

## Question 2:

A) Change in chronic management

If you are presented with an asthmatic patient with an acute exacerbation and *volume loss on x-ray* the explanation for the exacerbation is atelectasis and the proper management is a change in the chronic maintenance therapy.

# Case 23

(see page 75 for Questions)

Nail polish remover would suggest acetones and ketonemia

A 16 year-old girl with Type 1 diabetes since the age of 10 presents with severe abdominal pain and dry mouth. The smell of nail polish remover permeates the room so you look around but nobody has nail polish or appears to have recently removed the nail polish. The patient and parents insist that they follow a strict sliding scale regimen and are compliant.

Signs and symptoms consistent with DKA and dehydration

THE DIVERSION

Anything stated by patients or parents on the boards cannot be assumed to be true. In this case, despite claims to the contrary, one has to assume that there is poor compliance especially since the patient is a teenager.

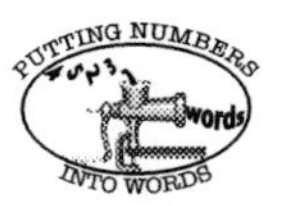


Acidosis, ketonuria, glucosuria, and marked hyper-glycemia

Her ABG reveals a pH of 7.29, serum glucose is 710 and her urine is positive for glucose and ketones.

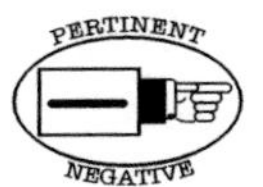


Guarding with no rebound makes an acute abdomen less likely especially given the other information in the vignette

Her physical exam is negative except for mild chest pain and abdominal pain with no guarding or rebound.

## Question 1:

D) NS Bolus 20 cc/KG

## Question 2:

B) Begin insulin drip 0.1 units/Kg/hour

## Question 3:

C) There is no correlation between low glycosylated hemoglobin levels and episodes of severe hypoglycemia

The *initial* management of DKA would be a normal saline fluid bolus. *Then,* an insulin drip should be started at 0.1 units/kg/hour. There is no increased incidence of severe hypoglycemia among patients with low glycosylated hemoglobin levels.

 

# Case 24

(see page 79 for Questions)

You are evaluating a 3-year-old girl with URI symptoms. During your examination you note that the patient has a lower than usual hairline with some facial asymmetry. The patient is developmentally delayed and the parents note that the child has a mild hearing deficit. Her neck has a decreased range of motion and appears to be shorter in proportion to the rest of the body with a webbed appearance. Cervical spine x-ray reveals fusion of cervical vertebrae 2 and 3.

Klippel-Feil Syndrome

Low hairline and facial asymmetry

Short neck

Fusion of cervical vertebrae

 

## Question 1:

D) Klippel-Feil Syndrome

## Question 2:

E) Cleft palate

The combination of fused cervical vertebrae, facial asymmetry, hearing deficit, low hairline and developmental delay is consistent with a diagnosis of Klippel-Feil syndrome.

Cleft palate is associated with Klippel-Feil syndrome and other associations include renal abnormalities, Sprengel deformity, hypermobility and congenital heart disease.

 

# Case 25

(see page 81 for Questions)

You are presented with a 6-week-old infant who, up until this point, has been a well-appearing, thriving infant. The baby was initially icteric on day 2 of life, which resolved without any intervention and the mother has continued to breast-feed. The infant was the product of a full-term gestation delivered by normal spontaneous vaginal delivery with Apgars of 9 and 9. There is no family history of liver disease.

The initial jaundice was probably physiologic jaundice and unrelated to the current condition.

The cause: something that can present at 6 weeks of age

On physical examination, the baby is noted to be well-nourished and in the 75th %ile for height, weight and head circumference. There are no obvious dysmorphic features. The baby is icteric including the sclerae and the rest of the exam is unremarkable.

Condition not associated with obvious dysmorphic features (ruling out Alagille syndrome)

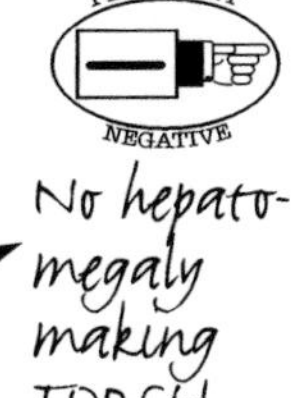


No hepatomegaly making TORCH less likely

(Continued on next page)

 

*(Continued from previous page)*

The serum indirect and direct bilirubin is 10.1/8.2

Increased direct and indirect bilirubin

## Question 1:

D) Biliary Atresia

## Question 2:

C) Abdominal ultrasound

## Question 3:

B) Liver Biopsy

The clinical picture presented is consistent with *biliary atresia.* The most appropriate next step to establish this diagnosis and distinguish it from other possible causes such as choledochal cyst would be abdominal *ultrasound.*

Keep in mind that a *liver* biopsy would be *more* definitive if included among the choices in distinguishing *intrahepatic cholestasis* from *biliary obstruction.* However, laparotomy and cholangiography would be the *most definitive.*

PERIL WARNING Remember, "jaundice" and "icterus" are exactly the same thing. We just tend to say "scleral icterus" and not "scleral jaundice" if the baby has icteric eyes. Do not get tripped up on the exam to think that icterus means the eyes are yellow unless it is specified. This is particularly important with children who are eating foods rich in beta-carotene who look yellow but are not icteric. In such a question they will make it a point to note that the eyes are not yellow.

Bottom line: Don't shoot for liver disease until you see the yellow in their eyes!

# Case 26

(see page 85 for Questions)

A 4-1/2 month old infant is brought to your office because the infant has not been himself, is lethargic, vomited twice last night and had a fever of 102.3 which was brought down to 100.1 with acetaminophen.

This is non specific and not helpful by itself

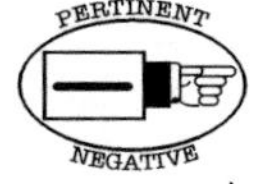


No diarrhea points away from viral gastro-enteritis

He has had not diarrhea. He has been around other children with a viral gastroenteritis.

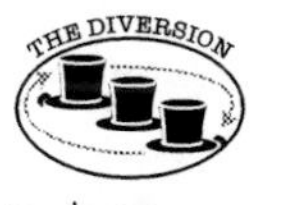


Physical examination shows a temperature of 101.5, respiratory rate of 25 and heart rate of 130 beats per minute. The baby seems to be very lethargic and difficult to console.

Inconsolability and lethargy would not be consistent with a garden-variety otitis or viral gastroenteritis.

HEENT – TM, red with decreased mobility and bulging on the right side. EOMI, PERRLA AF is full

Neck – supple, no meningismus

Bulging TM and negative meningismus is there to lead you to believe that meningitis is not the diagnosis.

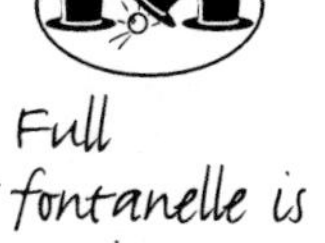


Full fontanelle is an important finding

(Continued on next page)

*(Continued from previous page)*

Lungs – clear

Card – S1 S2 no murmur, pulses 2+ throughout.

Abdomen – soft

Skin – no rashes noted

Neuro – symmetrical tone and strength

LABS

ANSWER REVEALED

CBC

WBC – 19.5 60 % neutrophils, 34% bands, 6% Lymphocytes

Leukocytosis is an important finding

H/H 9/36

*(Continued on next page)*

*(Continued from previous page)*

Lumbar Puncture:

Gram Stain –negative

Latex agglutination – negative

Glucose – 20

Protein- 80

Urinalysis – negative

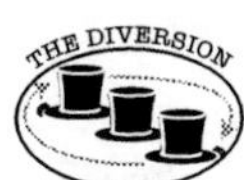


A negative LP does not rule out meningitis especially if the clinical findings suggest the diagnosis.

 

## Question 1:

E) Bacterial meningitis

## Question 2:

E) IV Vancomycin and Cefotaxime

Bulging TM and negative meningismus is there to lead you to believe that meningitis is not the diagnosis. However otitis media can indeed occur with meningitis especially in an infant. Negative meningismus in an infant in no way rules out meningitis.

A negative LP does not rule out meningitis especially if the clinical findings suggest the diagnosis, especially early. An LP performed 12 hours later could very likely reveal positive findings.

The most appropriate treatment would be IV Vancomycin to cover resistant *S. pneumoniae* and IV Cefotaxime to provide extended spectrum coverage.

The most likely etiological agents would include *Neisseria meningitidis*, *S. pneumoniae* and *Haemophilus influenza* although the latter would be the least likely due to the Hib vaccine over the past twenty years.

# Case 27

(see page 89 for Questions)

You are asked to evaluate a 6-week-old infant who a presents with inspiratory stridor and intercostal retractions. On physical examination you note that the child's cry is weak and the infant occasionally becomes cyanotic. The stridor has been present since birth.

Obstruction above the vocal cords, rules out tracheomalacia (expiratory distress) and unilateral vocal cord paralysis (hoarseness, breathy cough) and subglottic stenosis (biphasic stridor)

Sign of respiratory distress, rules out laryngomalacia

Consistent with a diagnosis of bilateral vocal cord paralysis

 

## Question 1:

A) Bilateral vocal cord paralysis

## Question 2:

D) Flexible upper airway endoscopy

This infant presents with congenital stridor. The most common cause of congenital stridor is laryngomalacia.

THE DIVERSION It is very easy to be fall into a pattern of believing that every time they present you with an infant with congenital stridor, especially inspiratory stridor, it is caused by laryngomalacia.

ANSWER REVEALED However, laryngomalacia does not present with signs of respiratory distress as this patient did. In fact, cyanotic spells and a weak cry in an infant presenting with congenital inspiratory stridor are more consistent with a diagnosis of bilateral vocal cord paralysis.

EITHER OR CHOICES **Subglottic stenosis** typically presents as biphasic stridor in an infant who has been intubated so watch for this description in the history.

**Unilateral vocal cord paralysis** would present as a breathy hoarse cry.

Bilateral vocal cord paralysis is best diagnosed by *flexible upper airway endoscopy.*

Microlaryngoscopy would be used to diagnosis subglottic stenosis.

Flexible or rigid bronchoscopy would be used to diagnose tracheomalacia.

Chest CT would be used to evaluate problems that are due to vascular anatomy of the chest, which is not the case with this patient.

 

# Case 28

(see page 91 for Questions)

You are called in by your obstetric colleague to evaluate a new rash on a woman who is at 39 weeks gestation. Of course, your colleagues call you in to evaluate rashes rather than the dermatologist because of your availability and much more favorable rates.

Would be funny if it were not true

You stroke your chin with your double gloved hand and look at the centrally umbilicated vesicular lesions concentrated on the trunk and their erythematous base; with several other similar lesions on the extremities, some of which are erythematous pruritic macules.

Classic description of chickenpox

 

## Question 1:

C) Chickenpox

## Question 2:

A) Dependent on the timing of the delivery

## Question 3:

A) Administer IM Varicella –zoster immunoglobulin to the baby

In this question you need to know that the mother has chickenpox. You also need to know that the newborn will only need treatment if the mother contracts the disease within 5 days prior to delivering or 2 days after delivering. (See *Laughing your way to Passing the Pediatric Boards® 3rd Edition* for a mnemonic that makes it impossible to forget this fact)

Therefore, the newborn will require treatment which consists of zoster immunoglobulin.

Please note that a vague diagnosis consisting of randomly aligned Latin terms such as "Macula-papular- eczematous pruritic non specific dermatitis" is the limited domain of the dermatology world. Ditto on the time buying "scrape and microscope viewing" maneuver described. This is the pediatric boards and such luxuries are not available and would be the incorrect choice.

 

# Case 29

(see page 95 for Questions)

Children with hemophilia typically injure the same joint

You are caring for a boy in your practice that repeatedly injures his right knee. Each injury results in a massive effusion and pain. After several negative orthopedic consults and MRIs you come across a pediatrician triple-boarded in pediatric EM, hematology and sports medicine who correctly diagnoses the problem as Hemophilia A. There is no family history of hemophilia.

Clinical description of hemarthroses

A little medical humor- something you probably won't see on the boards

THE DIVERSION

This is thrown in to confuse you into questioning the diagnosis. However, you need to know that hemophilia A can occur as a result of spontaneous mutation

## Question 1:

E) Female carriers can present with bleeding during pregnancy or surgery

## Question 2:

B) Soft tissue bleeding when they start crawling

## Question 3:

C) Factor 8 replacement at home

This vignette and series of questions is an opportunity to remember some important facts that will be very helpful on the exam:

- Factor activity of less than 1% results in spontaneous bleeding into joint spaces and soft tissue

INSIDER TIPS

**30% seems to be a popular number for Hemophilia and this fact alone should come in handy on the exam.**

- Hemophilia A can be the result of spontaneous mutation 30% of the time
- Female carriers who have a Factor 8 activity level of 30% will manifest with bleeding during surgery or pregnancy
- Only 30% of males with hemophilia A present with hemorrhage during circumcision

Factor 8 infusion is now largely home based

PERIL WARNING In this question if you did not know that hemophilia A was a result of Factor 8 deficiency you could easily have gotten a question like this wrong even if you knew treatment was home based.

 

# Case 30

(see page 99 for Questions)

Consistent history for chlamydia pneumonia. Recall the mnemonic:

Chlamydia
Cixteen weeks.

A 16-week-old afebrile infant presents with a runny nose and cough for the past 2 to 3 days. The baby has been breast fed with some supplementation. Breast-feeding has gone well. She was delivered by normal spontaneous vaginal delivery at full term with no complications. The prenatal course was unremarkable except for one time when the mother accidentally ate a piece mahi mahi maki sushi in Hawaii but spit most of it out on the floor several feet away on a surfer's booties. Group B strep cultures were negative and no intrapartum antibiotics were given.

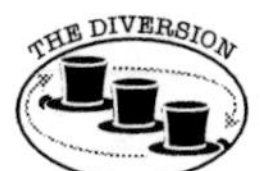


The eating of the sushi and the spitting on the surfer's booties is a diversion. Consuming raw fish during pregnancy, although not recommended, would not explain the symptoms in this infant.

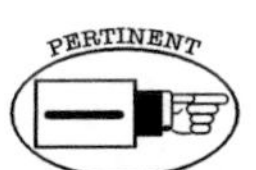


This helps rule out Group B strep pneumonia as the cause. In addition, Group B strep pneumonia would present with a much more toxic picture and a febrile infant

Physical examination shows that the infant has intercostal retractions and

(Continued on next page)

*(Continued from previous page)*

bilateral rales, with a respiratory rate of 52 breaths/min and a heart rate of 128 beats/min. Oxygen saturations are 96%. CXR shows diffuse infiltrates

PUTTING NUMBERS INTO WORDS

Tachypnea

## Question 1:

C) During the birth process

## Question 2:

D) Oral Azithromycin (Zithromax®)

The vignette is consistent with a diagnosis of chlamydia pneumonia. Since chlamydia is the etiology of the pneumonia it would have been acquired during the birth process. The most appropriate treatment in this case would be choice D, Oral Azithromycin (Zithromax®).

**Reference**

1. American Academy of Pediatrics. *Chlamydia (Chlamydophila)* pneumoniae. In: Pickering LK, ed. *American Academy of Pediatrics 2003 Report of the Committee on Infectious Diseases.* 26th ed. Elk Grove Village, Ill: American Academy of Pediatrics; 2003:325-237.

# Case 31

(see page 103 for Questions)

THE DIVERSION

These symptoms suggest renal etiology and can divert you into believing this is the correct workup leading to 3 incorrect answers in a row.

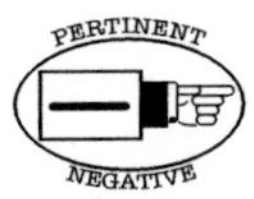


Afebrile, infectious etiology unlikely

A 14-year-old afebrile girl presents with acute onset of right lower quadrant tenderness with severe nausea and vomiting. The pain is sharp in nature and radiates to the back. She has not had dysuria, urgency, or diarrhea. The pain has been intermittent over the past 24 hours sometimes lasting 1-2 hours and then resolving spontaneously. Her last menstrual period was 3 weeks ago and she is sexually active but "always uses protection."

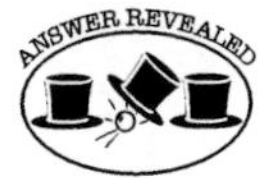


Intermittent pain wold suggests a process that is not constant, that twists and untwists. Right sided adnexal pain suggests pain is ovarian in origin although ectopic pregnancy is a possibility

On physical exam she is in considerable pain with vital signs within normal limits. Her abdomen is soft but tender with no guarding or rebound tenderness.

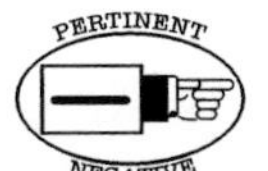


The absence of rebound points away from appendicitis or obstruction

(Continued on next page)

*(Continued from previous page)*

The abdominal pain is increased over the right lower quadrant.

Bowel sounds are present. Bimanual exam reveals right sided adnexal tenderness with no increased cervical motion tenderness

Intermittent pain wold suggests a process that is not constant, that twists and untwists. Right sided adnexal pain suggests pain is ovarian in origin although ectopic pregnancy is a possibility

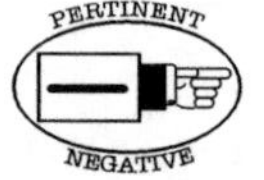


RBC in urine suggests the possibility of a renal stone

CBC – WBC- 9.5 with a normal differential

Na/ 139 K / 4.0 Cl/ 105 Glucose/ 95 Bun/ 15 Cre/ 0.3 Bicarb/ 24

Urinalysis – negative except for 20 RBC

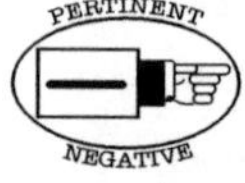


Urine HCG – Negative

Negative HCG rules out pregnancy.

## Question 1:

A) Abdominal CT

## Question 2:

D) Ovarian Torsion

## Question 3:

B) Laparoscopic exploration

Abrupt onset of pain which is colicky in nature and radiates to the back is typical of ovarian torsion. In fact it is quite similar to the colicky pain of a renal stone. Therefore an abdominal CT scan would help make the diagnosis. Likewise an ectopic pregnancy can also present in a similar fashion.

If the urine HCG is negative it is unlikely that the serum Beta Quant will be positive. IVP won't be helpful in establishing the diagnosis. Since the physical findings and history suggest an ovarian torsion an abdominal CT would be most helpful in establishing the diagnosis.

Laparoscopic exploration would be the most logical therapeutic intervention and if indicated untwisting of the ovary. Salpingo-oophorectomy would be indicated if necrotic tissue is present but *at this time* it would not be the correct intervention. *Oophoropexy* of the uninvolved ovary (basically anchoring it) may be indicated and would be a correct answer if it were included among different choices.

# Case 32

(see page 107 for Questions)

An 8-year-old boy presents with a patchy distribution of hair loss over the past 8 weeks. On physical exam you note 2 areas of hair loss in the frontal region of the scalp that are complete, with the exposed skin appearing smooth. There are no broken hairs noted and no erythema. The rest of the physical exam is unremarkable except for nail pitting.

Classic description of alopecia areata

Nail pitting can be seen with alopecia areata

## Question 1:

C) Alopecia areata

## Question 2:

E) Reassurance

Alopecia areata will be described as appearing in the frontal or parietal scalp as smooth and non-erythematous with no broken hairs noted. Nail pitting can also be seen. The majority will grow hair within one year, therefore, nothing beyond reassurance is needed.

# Case 33

(see page 109 for Questions)

An 18-year-old female returns from winter break complaining of palpitations and difficulty sleeping as well as weight loss and decreased appetite. On physical examination you notice a tremor in both of her hands and her eyes seem to be more pronounced than you would like. She is also unable to tolerate heat and sleeps with the windows opened even when it is below freezing outside. There is a symmetrical non-tender mass over her anterior neck. She was a straight "A" student in high school and has been struggling to get C's in college. She is taking no medications and her urine tox screen and pregnancy test are both negative.

Non specific findings demonstrating anxiety

Exophthalmia

THE DIVERSION

These are findings that are also consistent with hypothyroid but none of the other findings are.

Enlarged thyroid

Non specific

## Question 1:

C) Serum T3, T4, and TSH levels

## Question 2:

E) Graves disease

## Question 3:

E) Thyroid ablation

The history is fairly non –specific and could be consistent with a diagnosis of bipolar mood disorder, pheochromocytoma or Addison's disease to some degree. However the description of thyroid enlargement and exophthalmia points only to Graves disease as the correct diagnosis and Serum T3, T4, and TSH levels as the appropriate tests to order. Graves disease is treated by thyroid ablation which could come in the form of medication (methimazole, carbimazole or propylthiouracil, Surgical or with $I^{131}$).

# Case 34

(see page 111 for Questions)

A 12-year-old girl presents because of a severe cough that has kept her up at night and out of school for the past 3 days. She had the flu including high fever, vomiting and diarrhea and cough. All but the cough symptoms have resolved. The mother notes that she has had "chronic bronchitis" since she was a child. In the past, Azithromycin has worked wonders. Fortunately she had an extra pack in one of the shoeboxes in her shoe closet but it has not helped this time. She would like you to treat the bronchitis this time.

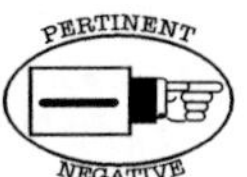


Nightime cough which keeps her up at night. This rules out psychogenic cough

Cough following a viral illness after it has resolved.

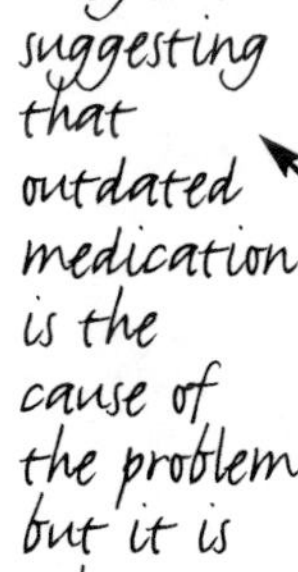

They are suggesting that outdated medication is the cause of the problem but it is only a diversion or an illusion designed to take you off the trail.

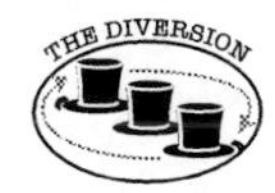


Chronic bronchitis is in quotes suggesting an incorrect diagnosis.

## Question 1:

D) Bronchospasm

## Question 2:

D) Albuterol via metered dose inhaler

## Question 3:

E) Oral prednisone for 5 days

A severe cough following a viral illness that keeps the patient up at night should suggest reactive airway disease as the correct diagnosis. If the correct diagnosis was psychogenic cough they would have noted that the cough resolves while the patient is asleep.

Any diagnosis in quotes is most likely the incorrect diagnosis. Typically, bronchitis or pneumonia in quotes suggests asthma or reactive airway disease as the correct diagnosis.

# Case 35

(see page 113 for Questions)

A 14-year-old girl complains of recurrent headaches, which are throbbing and pulsating in nature and felt most severely behind her right eye. She is a competitive cross country skier and the headaches are most severe when she is training the hardest or otherwise exerting herself physically. She experiences no muscle cramping with the headaches. The headaches are usually accompanied by waves of nausea and vomiting. She is meticulous with rehydrating during training consistent with training protocol confirmed by her trainer. The only relief for her headaches is lying down and sleeping in a quiet room with the lights dimmed. She has avoided seeking medical attention because of fears she will be told to quit skiing and

Consistent with a vascular/migraine headache

Headaches worsened with physical exertion

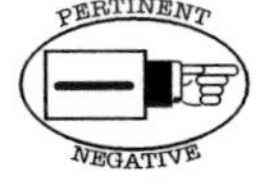


Potassium wasting not a likely factor

*(Continued on next page)*

 

(Continued from previous page)

with a college scholarship in the wings this is not an option. She has also taken no medications fearing this would disqualify her from Olympic trials.

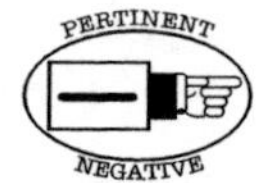


Performance enhancing steroids unlikely

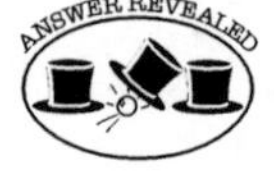


She is popular with friends and has maintained her grades despite the increasing frequency of her headaches. You obtain a urine HCG, which is negative and her last menstrual period was 2 weeks ago and has been regular.

Points away from Pulmonary cause Cardiology is a possibility but with the absence of a murmur and no clinical improvement, makes it unlikely

Eating disorder unlikely

PHYSICAL EXAM:

General – well nourished female with weight and height in the 60th percentile for age
HEENT – no evidence of papilledema, EOMI, PERRLA
SMR (Tanner) – 3

(Continued on next page)

*(Continued from previous page)*

Lungs – clear

Card – S1, S2 no murmur, normal sinus rhythm, cap refill less than 2 seconds

Abd- soft, non-tender

## Question 1:

C) Head CT

## Question 2:

C) Migraine headaches

## Question 3:

C) Ibuprofen and close followup

A headache that is *throbbing, unilateral, retroorbital, worsened with physical exertion and relieved with sleep in a lightly dimmed room* is consistent with a diagnosis of a migraine headache.

PERIL WARNING However, since she has not sought any medical attention in the past, no imaging studies have been performed. Since migraine headaches are a diagnosis of exclusion one must first obtain a head CT.

INSIDER TIPS Steroid use is unlikely in this patient as are any drugs that may be detected in a tox screen. The most appropriate fluid replacement in teenage athletes is plain water, not water with salt pills. Since she isn't experiencing muscular cramps hypokalemia is unlikely as is the need for potassium supplements during training.

 

# Case 36

(see page 117 for Questions)

A 12-year-old girl appears at your office on a Friday at 5:05 PM (for her 3:30 PM one Wednesday) in the cold and dark of December. Her mother tells you that the girl has been limping for a couple of weeks because of severe left-sided knee pain. Her past medical history is negative except for continued weight gain despite several attempts to lose weight with the help of a nutritionist. They live in a wooded area and she has not traveled recently.

She has been afebrile, and does not recall being hit in the knee or leg. She is taking no medications and has not had any recent viral illnesses. She has difficulty moving her leg inward.

Age, left sided referred knee pain, and difficulty with inward rotation are classic signs of SCFE

Overweight, another classic component of SCFE

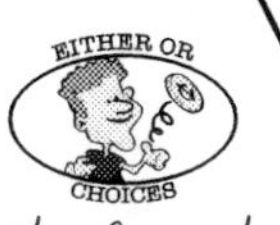


The fact that she is afebrile points away from septic arthritis, osteomyelitis and other infectious etiologies

Points away from a traumatic etiology

Negative past medical history would include a negative history of sickle cell disease making aseptic necrosis of hip an unlikely diagnosis.

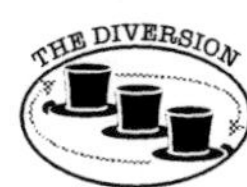


This information is placed to divert you into believing that this is due to lyme arthritis. However, early in the question it is noted that this is a cold and dark December when one is unlikely to contract lyme disease

No recent viral illnesses points away from post viral synovitis

Age, left sided referred knee pain, and difficulty with inward rotation are classic signs of SCFE

 

## Question 1:

B) anteroposterior and frog lateral x-rays of the pelvis

## Question 2:

E) Slipped capital femoral epiphysis left hip

## Question 3:

C) Surgical correction

Slipped capital femoral epiphysis typically presents in girls aged 11 to 13 years and boys aged 13 to 15 years who are obese. Although race was not noted in this question, it is more common in black patients than in white. Although a slipped capital femoral epiphysis can produce pain localized to the groin area, it often presents as knee pain, especially on the board examination. Internal rotation is difficult. If you were to suggest an x-ray, anteroposterior and frog lateral x-rays of the pelvis would be the way to go.

**Reference**

1. Loder RT, Richards BS, Shapiro PS, et al. Acute slipped capital epiphysis: the importance of physeal stability. *J Bone Joint Surg Am.* 1993;75A:1134-1140

# Case 37

(see page 119 for Questions)

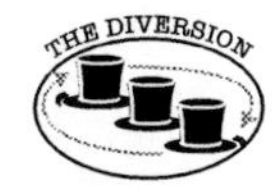


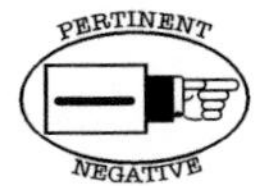


You are evaluating an afebrile 15-year-old girl with severe abdominal pain and vomiting but no diarrhea. The pain has occurred over the past 2 days and radiates to her back. She has remained afebrile and has not changed her diet nor has she traveled out of the U.S. recently. The pain is severe and intermittent and has interfered with her sleep although she can sleep once the pain subsides. On physical examination the pain is primarily in the right upper quadrant. There is no significant family history of any GI disease.

This is thrown in to lead to you to the misdiagnosis of pancreatitis or pyelonephritis

Makes cholecystitis unlikely

Intermittent colicky pain points to a gallstone

Gallbladder pain

## Question 1:

E) Abdominal ultrasound

## Question 2:

B) Cholelithiasis

## Question 3:

D) Cholecystectomy

The combination of intermittent colicky right upper quadrant pain all but hand-feeds you a diagnosis of cholelithiasis (or gallstones as they are known in normal non-medical circles). The most specific and sensitive (and not to mention least invasive) test to diagnose cholelithiasis would be an abdominal ultrasound.

While pancreatitis can be a secondary complication, primary pancreatitis is unlikely to be the cause of the symptoms this patient is experiencing. Therefore amylase/lipase would not be helpful in establishing a diagnosis and the next step would not be ERCP.

Cholecystectomy would be the treatment of choice in this situation.

# Case 38

*(see page 121 for Questions)*

Low grade fever

Acute Otalgia does not automatically mean otitis media

A 3-year-old girl presents with a fever of 100.2°F and severe ear pain. It is a Saturday morning and you are covering for their regular pediatrician, Dr. Treatemall. According to the parents, "this happens all the time," with this being the 3rd episode in 6 weeks. The child's aunt, who up until now was quietly sending text messages in the corner, blurts out "Dr. Treatemall always gives us the pink medicine and sometimes the white fruity one except for that one time he gave us the yellow tutti-fruity ones which were the only samples he had left in his pocket!"

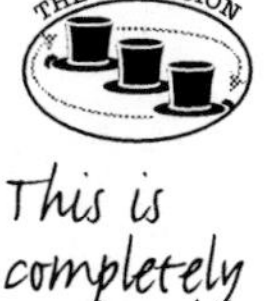


This is completely within the normal range for age and would not in any way indicate an immunology workup

On Physical exam, the child is afebrile with stable vital signs. Respiratory rate is 32 and unlabored.

Non Toxic child

*(Continued on next page)*

 

(Continued from previous page)

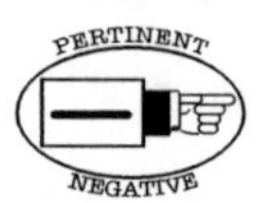


Benign physical findings

The child is alert, with some discomfort, nasal congestion, and slight cough. Lungs on auscultation are clear, no rales, wheeze or rhonchi. Cardiac exam reveals S1 S2, normal sinus rhythm, pulses 2+ throughout with cap refill < 2 seconds.

Her tympanic membranes are red, with positive movement on insufflation. The tympanogram does show a peaked curve.

THE DIVERSION

Normal mobility and tympanogram curve which is inconsistent with acute otitis media

PERIL

WARNING

A red TM does not automatically make for a diagnosis of otitis media especially on the boards. You don't expect it to be that easy do you?

## Question 1:

E) No diagnostic studies are indicated at this point

## Question 2:

B) Acetaminophen

The clinical vignette described is typical of myringitis, or inflammation of the tympanic membrane, but not of otitis media (OM). Therefore, antibiotic treatment would not be indicated. In OM, you would expect blunting of the curve on tympanogram, and insufflation would reveal *decreased mobility*. In addition, with OM, we would expect a more ill appearing child. Decongestants or antihistamines have no proven value in treating myringitis or OM. Acetaminophen will help alleviate the pain and is the only medication indicated for this patient.

**Reference**

1. Siegel RM, Kiely M, Bien JP, et al. Treatment of otitis media with observation and a safety-net antibiotic prescription. *Pediatrics.* 2003;112:527-531.

 

# Case 39

(see page 125 for Questions)

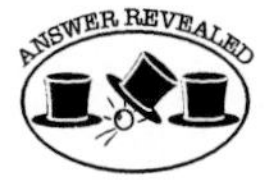


Over 3 months

You are evaluating a 7-year-old boy who has had bouts of excruciating abdominal pain for well over a year. The parents are besides themselves and have had their son evaluated by a nutritionist, herbologist, homeopathic doctor and even a pediatric gastroenterologist at the university medical center. Despite a "boatload of tests" done by all of these consultants, the pain continues. The pain is worse in September and seems to get better during the summer and during winter and spring break.

Organic disease has been ruled out

Emotional component, increases during stressful times, decreases during more relaxed times

PERTINENT NEGATIVE

Normal Growth points away from inflammatory bowel disease

He has had no weight loss and is at the 60th percentile for weight and height. He has experienced intermittent headaches with the belly pain and some nausea but no diarrhea or constipation. Stool is heme negative and has been normal in size and color.

Consistent with recurrent functional abdominal pain

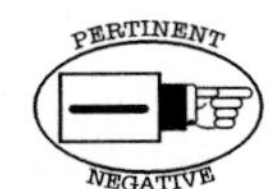


Rules out celiac sprue

## Question 1:

D) Functional recurrent abdominal pain

## Question 2:

E) Reassurance and counseling

## Question 3:

E) Symptoms will continue into adulthood in up to 50% of patients

The patient in the vignette is presenting with classic *functional recurrent abdominal pain* aka irritable bowel syndrome, which can also present with nausea and headaches.

By noting that the child has already been seen by a GI specialist despite the red herring herbologist and homeopath thrown in for good measure they are telling you that the patient has all organic disease ruled out. This fact coupled with their noting that the pain increases during stressful times and decreases during non-stressful times leaves only one diagnostic possibility and that is functional recurrent abdominal pain.

Up to 50% of children with this will continue to have symptoms into adulthood. The best treatment is reassurance and psychological counseling.

# Case 40

(see page 127 for Questions)

A 2-year-old presents with a 4-day history of cough and respiratory distress and chest tightness, which has gotten progressively worse.

Non specific findings

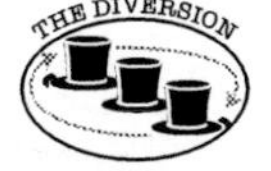


Father's smoking and aspiration of foreign body are possible. Need to read the rest of the findings to determine if this is real or a diversion.

Except for 2 episodes of post tussive emesis he has had no vomiting or diarrhea. The parents are careful to keep choking hazards out of reach and do not believe he ingested or aspirated any foreign bodies. The father smokes but always in a different room or outside.

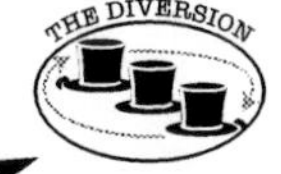


His past history is significant for 3 episodes of lobar pneumonia, twice requiring hospitalization. You look up his medical records from his previous admissions and note that both times he had pneumonia involving the right lower lobe.

Recurrent pneumonia involving the same lobe suggests an anatomical abnormality

(Continued on next page)

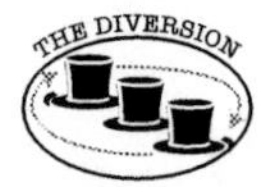

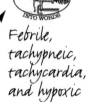

Recurrent pneumonia involving the same lobe suggests an anatomical abnormality

(Continued from previous page)

He was born at 37 weeks gestation and was large for gestational age. The delivery was traumatic with Apgars of 4 at one minute and 9 at 5 minutes. He was in the NICU for 4 days and required some supplemental oxygen. There was decreased movement of his right arm diagnosed as Erb's palsy but with some physical therapy his range of motion is almost fully recovered.

On physical exam he is in moderate distress breathing at 75 breaths / minute, heart rate is 165, with an oxygen saturation of 90% in room air. He has a temperature of 101.2.

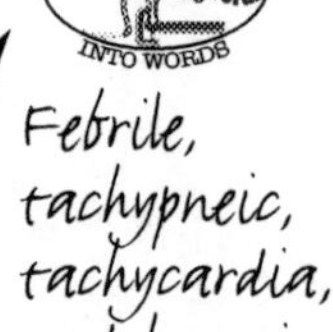


Febrile, tachypneic, tachycardia, and hypoxic

(Continued on next page)

*(Continued from previous page)*

His lungs are clear but there are significant subcostal and intercostal retractions with nasal flaring. There are decreased breath sounds on the right side.

CXR – right lower lobe infiltrate as well as elevation of the right hemidiaphragm

Respiratory distress, Right sided process

## Question 1:

A) Real Time Fluoroscopy

## Question 2:

B) IV Ceftriaxone

## Question 3:

E) Referral to Pediatric Surgery

The cause of this child's problem is *diaphragmatic paralysis* due to a phrenic nerve injury during birth trauma. This is indeed associated with an Erb's Palsy which should be the revelation buried in the question. Another association to keep in mind for children with a history of birth trauma is *Horner syndrome* presenting as *ptosis* and *miosis.*[1]

The recurrent pneumonia involving the same lobe should suggest an anatomical cause of the pneumonia. The history of Erb's Palsy should suggest diaphragmatic paralysis automatically. This alone should allow you to pick the correct answer. The immediate intervention would be the same regardless of the underlying problem. The child has pneumonia on x-ray and needs to be treated with IV antibiotics.

EITHER OR CHOICES Foreign body aspiration is a possibility even though the parents did not notice the child swallowing any foreign objects and keeping choking hazards out of reach. The father's smoking is not helpful but in this case not relevant. The history does not suggest a diagnosis of RSV pneumonia or asthma.

---

[1] Which is pinpoint pupils. See *Laughing your way to Passing the Pediatric Boards®* for a mnemonic to help distinguish miosis from mydriasis in an instant.

# Case 41

(see page 131 for Questions)

This is most likely physiologic jaundice and unrelated to the cause of the jaundice at this age.

You are evaluating a 7-month-old infant who has become increasingly jaundiced over the past few weeks. With the exception of mild hyperbilirubinemia during the initial postnatal days, the baby has not been jaundiced at all. The mother's blood type is A+ and the baby is O negative. The baby has been not been gaining weight adequately since 2 months of age. On physical examination you note wide spaced eyes and a smaller than usual mandible.

No ABO incompatibility

THE DIVERSION

The small mandible might have diverted you into believing Pierre Robin syndrome is the diagnosis.

Failure to thrive since age 2 months

On physical exam the baby is icteric. Lungs are clear and the cardiac exam is normal except for a grade 3/6 murmur.

PUTTING NUMBERS INTO WORDS

Cardiac disease

The total and direct bilirubin is 7.6/5.5

PUTTING NUMBERS INTO WORDS

Indirect and direct hyperbilirubinemia

## Question 1:

B) Alagille Syndrome

## Question 2:

A) Marked hepatomegaly

## Question 3:

D) 70% with liver transplantation

In infants with Alagille syndrome (aka arteriohepatic dysplasia, the most common form of familial intrahepatic cholestasis), bile ducts are lost progressively during infancy resulting in failure to thrive and the gradual onset of symptoms.

Dysmorphic features are important components including a small mandible. However the other signs are not consistent with a diagnosis of Pierre Robin syndrome.

INSIDER TIPS If you are presented with an infant with dysmorphic features who becomes icteric later in infancy you should think of Alagille syndrome

Additional findings in Alagille syndrome include:

- Hyperlipidemia
- Cutaneous xanthomas
- Vertebral anomalies
- Anomalies of the eye
- Anomalies of the kidney (less common)

PERIL WARNING Hepatomegaly is *frequently* but *not always* present in Alagille syndrome.

# Case 42

(see page 133 for Questions)

A 2-year-old boy is brought to your office because of persistent high fever despite being given ibuprofen every 8 hours as suggested on the bottle. He was seen in the emergency room when the fever started one week ago and was given amoxicillin for an ear infection.

The past medical history is non – contributory. He attends day care with 3 other boys who are all in good health according to the mother.

She is very frustrated because the child has been miserable, complaining of a belly-ache and that his legs hurt. She wants you to "take care of this infection".

THE DIVERSION

These are diversions to lead you to believe that the diagnosis is due to a strep infection or other etiology

These are findings consistent with a diagnosis of Kawasaki disease

(Continued on next page)

*(Continued from previous page)*

PHYSICAL EXAM-

T 39.5 HR 180 RR 55

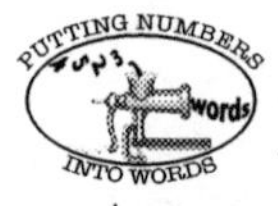


High fever for several days, tachycardia and tachypnea (consistent with high fever)

General – The boy appears to be irritable and very uncomfortable
HEENT – TM non-injected with good mobility, conjunctiva are injected with no exudate
Throat – mild erythema but difficult to examine, oral mucosa and lips are dry with some cracking of the skin on the lips

Neck – Supple, + palpable anterior cervical lymph nodes which are firm on exam
Card – S1 S2, No murmur
Skin – Positive Rash, which is raised but blanches well

Extremities- non-pitting edema of the hands and feet

These are findings consistent with a diagnosis of Kawasaki disease

*(Continued on next page)*

*(Continued from previous page)*

LABS-

Rapid Strep- negative

Mono Spot-negative

Blood Culture Pending

CBC –

WBC – 15.6

60 % Neutrophils, 30% Lymphocytes

Platelet Count – 420 → Thrombocytosis

H/H – 32/11.5

Erythrocyte sedimentation rate- 55 mm/h → Elevated ESR

LFT

ALT level is 100 U/L

AST, 295 U/L

Alkaline phosphatase, 171 U/L

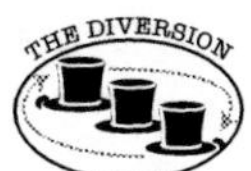


Cardiac Echo – unremarkable → The normal cardiac echo does not rule out Kawasaki in any way since this is typically a later finding

 

## Question 1:

A) IVIG 2g/Kg

## Question 2:

E) Unknown

The child in this vignette meets the criteria of fever lasting 5 days and at least four criteria of Kawasaki disease:

1) Bilateral non exudative conjunctivitis
2) Injected fissured lips
3) Injected Pharynx
4) Edema of hands and feet
5) Cervical adenopathy

Therefore, a presumptive diagnosis of Kawasaki disease can be made. Therefore, the most important next step in management would be IVIG. IVIG reduces both the duration of fever and the prevalence of coronary artery aneurysm when given within 10 days of onset. However, there is no documented etiology of Kawasaki–just theories. The use of steroids is controversial and therefore would not be the correct choice. In addition, acetylsalicylic acid PO would be appropriate treatment to prevent coronary artery disease; however, acetaminophen would not be.

# Case 43

(see page 137 for Questions)

Preceding URI

A 3-year-old girl presents with a one-week history of cough and rhinorrhea and a new temperature of 103.9°F. Today she has developed increased respiratory distress along with expiratory stridor that is quite frightening to the parents and her cough is now brassy and productive. A chest x-ray reveals patchy infiltrate and an atypical tracheal air column. The child's immunization status is up to date and she has otherwise been healthy.

Febrile

Secretions and expiratory stridor

Patchy infiltrates and atypical tracheal air column consistent with a diagnosis of Bacterial tracheitis

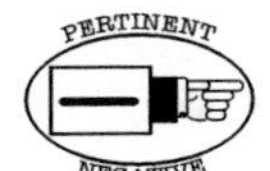


Rules out asthma and H. Flu epiglottitis

## Question 1:

A) Bronchoscopy to clear secretions and antibiotic coverage for Staph aureus

## Question 2:

D) Bacterial tracheitis

Bacterial tracheitis typically occurs in a child who is age 3 or younger, usually preceded by a viral URI. This then leads to high fever and dyspnea followed by expiratory stridor followed by copious thick purulent discharge.

This is typically caused by *Staph aureus* and the immediate treatment is clearing of the copious secretions followed by antibiotic coverage for *Staph aureus.*

Asthma and H. Flu epiglottitis are ruled out. Therefore intubation in the OR is not indicated. This is also not a typical picture of viral croup and therefore racemic epinephrine and dexamethasone are not indicated.

THE DIVERSION

Noting that the cough is *brassy* is a diversionary tactic to lead you to believe that viral croup is the etiology.

# Case 44

(see page 139 for Questions)

PERTINENT NEGATIVE

Afebrile infectious etiology unlikely

You are seeing an afebrile 6-year-old boy in the emergency department with a 2-day history of cough and rhinorrhea. His parents report that he is coughing a lot but can't seem to "cough up any mucous" resulting in coughing spasms. In the ER you note that his cough is weak. In the afternoon, he has a difficult time opening his eyes, although this does not seem to be a problem in the morning when he wakes up. On the weekends he is able to walk around and play with other children but he poops out in the early afternoon and hangs out with adults.

Non specific findings

This would suggest chest wall muscle weakness

ANSWER REVEALED

Weakness which worsens as the day progresses is suggestive of myasthenia gravis

His past medical history is unremarkable and his immunizations are up to date.

(Continued on next page)

 

*(Continued from previous page)*

On physical exam he is an alert, responsive boy. He has a difficult time speaking, swallows with difficulty and has diminished gag reflex. EOMI, PERRLA, bilateral ptosis.

Bulbar muscle weakness

His lungs are clear without wheezing, rales or rhonchi. His neurological exam is remarkable for decreased strength in all 4 extremities with normal deep tendon reflexes.

Muscle weakness is consistent with myasthenia gravis but by itself non-specific

CXR – clear with no infiltrates

CBC – WBC 6.5 with a normal differential

Blood Culture pending

## Question 1:

D) Edrophonium test

## Question 2:

D) Myasthenia Gravis

## Question 3:

B) Pyridostigmine

The clinical findings and presentation in this vignette are consistent with a diagnosis of **myasthenia gravis**, which is due to the destruction of acetylcholine receptors by an antibody that targets these receptors. Weakness and fatigability that increases as the day progresses are classic findings. Coupled with the bulbar musculature weakness in this patient, it nails the diagnosis.

**Guillain Barré** syndrome would present with an ascending paralytic pattern. **Botulism** usually occurs in infants and would also present with decreased deep tendon reflexes. Transverse myelitis and Lyme have markedly different presenting signs and symptoms.

Edrophonium is an anticholinesterase inhibitor, which is a double negative. Bottom-line it increases the amount of acetylcholine in the receptor and symptomatic relief is seen immediately, albeit briefly. This helps establish the diagnosis and is commonly known as the Tensilon® test.

Pharmacological treatment of myasthenia gravis is with pyridostigmine.

# Case 45

(see page 143 for Questions)

You are asked to consult on a 9-month-old boy who presents with respiratory distress.

Past medical history is positive for recurrent otitis media. The baby was born by spontaneous vaginal delivery, which was uneventful. The mother's prenatal care is unknown.

The fact that they point out the recurrent OM is significant and should be noted and make you consider an immunodeficiency

The mother's unknown history is an important point. They would not mention it if it wasn't important. In fact, you should assume inadequate prenatal care or an undiagnosed disorder in the mother

PHYSICAL EXAM:

Afebrile, RR 55, Oxygen Saturations 88-91% on room air.

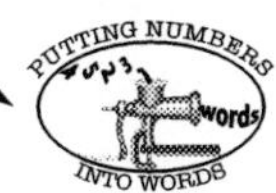


Tachypnea and hypoxia

Weight – Below the 5th percentile for age.

Failure to thrive

HEENT- EOMI, PERRLA, Ears with scarring on TMs bilaterally. Throat clear

(Continued on next page)

*(Continued from previous page)*

Neck – Supple, positive cervical adenopathy

Lungs – Clear

Abdomen- Liver palpable 4 cm below the costal margin with a palpable spleen

Hepatosplenomegaly

CXR- Hyperinflation and bilateral perihilar infiltrates with no consolidation noted.

X-ray findings consistent with Pneumocystis carinii

## Question 1:

A) Hypergammaglobulinemia

## Question 2:

E) The diagnosis of *Pneumocystis carinii* is confirmed by bronchioalveolar lavage (BAL)

Hypergammaglobulinemia is consistent with a diagnosis of HIV infection. The elevated immunoglobulins are not helpful in fighting infection since they are mostly hypofunctioning. In addition, the following would also be consistent with a diagnosis of HIV infection

- Leukopenia
- Thrombocytopenia
- Low CD4/CD8 ratio
- Elevated alanine aminotransferase level

The diagnosis of Pneumocystis carinii is confirmed by *bronchioalveolar lavage.* Prophylaxis with Trimethoprim-Sulfamethoxazole is done once CD4 lymphocytes suppression is severe as outlined by the CDC and not immediately upon diagnosis. **Successful treatment with Ceftriaxone does not rule out disease.**

THE DIVERSION Polymerase chain reaction is how HIV infection is confirmed, not how *Pneumocystis Carinii* is confirmed.

Varicella vaccine should be given to HIV infected patients who have normal CD4+ levels.

 

# Case 46

(see page 147 for Questions)

You are asked to evaluate a 4-year-old boy who was diagnosed with ADHD last year. He was started on methylphenidate 5 mg a day, which has not improved his behavior. His parents claim that he is a "very anxious child". You notice that he speaks in a high pitched tone, repeats a lot of the same phrases and is very playful. His attention span is short even when factoring in his age.

A diagnosis of ADHD prior to age 7 would be inappropriate. All choices related to ADHD will be incorrect.

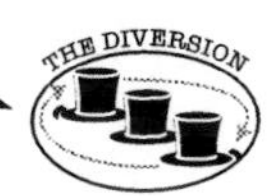


This is a diversion to lead you to believe the diagnosis is William Syndrome

On physical exam you note that his head circumference is > 95th%ile with thickened nasal bridge, protruding ears and an elongated face and pointed chin, simian creases are noted on both hands and his testicles are unusually large with an SMR of 1.

These are classic physical findings consistent with Fragile X syndrome

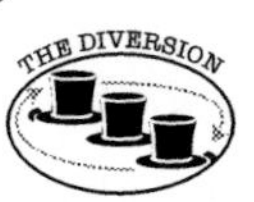


The simian crease is noted to try to divert you into believing the correct diagnosis is Down Syndrome.

## Question 1:

C) Fragile X Syndrome

## Question 2:

B) Molecular genetic analysis

## Question 3:

D) Multidisciplinary management and care

The physical findings are classic findings of Fragile X syndrome[1] Standard Karyotyping will not help in making the correct diagnosis of Fragile X. Only very specific *genetic molecular analysis* (way to boring to get into here) will reveal the "fragility of the X chromosome" in question.

Methylphenidate and atomoxetine would be appropriate treatments for ADHD but this is not the correct diagnosis in the patient. There is not definitive treatment for Fragile X, only multidisciplinary management of specific medical and behavioral challenges.

A simian crease can be present in Fragile X syndrome as well. In can also be seen in individuals with no syndrome at all.

[1] See our companion Laughing your way to passing the Pediatric Boards® for the celebrity with similar features.

 

# Case 47

(see page 149 for Questions)

A Caucasian 6-week-old boy is brought in because of severe dehydration that has gotten progressively worse over the past 3 days.

Severe dehydration out of proportion with the degree of diarrhea seen.

He weighs approximately one pound less than his birth weight and has developed non-bloody diarrhea.

Failure to thrive

The diarrhea has no mucous and is normal in appearance and texture. The infant has remained afebrile with no vomiting although at 10 days of life he was switched to a soy based formula because of loose stools and 2 episodes of vomiting.

Difficulty with formula early on

There is no family history of any metabolic disorders. He is currently on soy formula. The birth history is unremarkable.

(Continued on next page)

*(Continued from previous page)*

PUTTING NUMBERS INTO WORDS

Tachypnea and tachycardia

On physical exam the baby is lethargic, somewhat hypotonic and cyanotic with a shrill cry that makes the entire department's hair stand on end. He appears to be cachectic. He is afebrile with a HR of 180, respiratory rate of 65, and BP of 86/35. His weight is below the 5%ile for age. His pulse oximetry is 85% and does not improve with supplemental oxygen.

Points away from Pulmonary cause. Cardiac cause is a possibility but with the absence of a murmur and no clinical improvement, makes it unlikely

HEENT- dry mucous membranes, flat anterior fontanelle with sunken eyes and poor tear production while crying

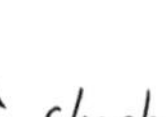


Lungs- Clear with nasal flaring and mild respiratory distress

Card – S1 S2 no murmur, weak peripheral pulses with a cap refill of 3-4 seconds

*(Continued on next page)*

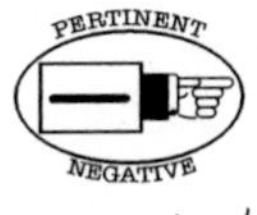


*(Continued from previous page)*

Abdomen- soft, non-tender, no hepatomegaly

GU- normal male genitalia with both testes descended

Congenital adrenal hyperplasia very unlikely

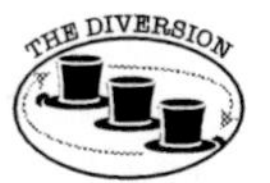


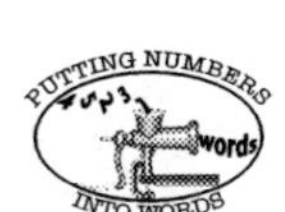


LABS-

CBC- WBC – 19.5, 20% Neutrophils 10% bands 40% lymphocytes
Lytes, Na/ 129, K/5.0 Cl/109 Bicarb/15
Bun/ 30 Cre/0.4 Glucose/ 110
Blood Culture sent

Hyponatremia and acidosis would be consistent with dehydration and are general signs

The high WBC with left shift might trick you into believing the ultimate diagnosis is sepsis. This can be seen with any illness

Lumbar puncture-no evidence of spinal meningitis
RSV- negative

Rules out RSV bronchiolitis

CXR- no consolidation or cardiomegaly
ABG- although the sample was drawn from the radial artery the blood appeared to be venous, even brown in color
pH 7.21/ CO2 18/ O2/ 200

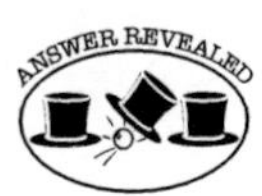


Most revealing and suggestive

 

## Question 1:

C) IV antibiotics and normal saline bolus

## Question 2:

E) Methemoglobinemia

## Question 3:

C) Methylene blue

The most revealing part of the history is "blood appeared to be venous, even brown in color" which is suggestive of the correct diagnosis of methemoglobinemia. However any lethargic infant with signs of shock should be assumed to be septic until proven otherwise and therefore the *initial step* should include IV antibiotics and fluids.

No increase in oxygen saturation despite supplemental oxygen would be consistent with congenital cardiac disease however one would expect *some clinical improvement.* However this does make pulmonary disease unlikely. Combined with the negative RSV, pulmonary disease is essentially ruled out.

Methemoglobinemia should be considered in the differential of any toxic-appearing infant presenting with cyanosis, diarrhea and shock. Watch for cyanosis that does not respond to supplemental oxygen and the blood is darker than expected. One of the most important signs will be an infant with diarrhea whose toxic appearance is out of proportion with the presenting history.

---

**Reference:** An infant with methemoglobinemia, Nelson and Hostetler, Hospital Physician, February 2003 62:31-38

# Case 48

(see page 153 for Questions)

You are evaluating a new patient to your practice that is 4 months old. He was born in Honduras and just arrived in the U.S. last month. His birth history is unknown and his medical records are unknown. On physical exam you note that the sutures are widely separated and the patient has a protruding tongue and coarse facial features. The rest of the physical exam is unremarkable except for an umbilical hernia, which is easily reducible.

Born outside US in developing country, consider: undiagnosed chronic disease, disease screened for in U.S. or disease for which immunization is available in the U.S.

Separated sutures

Despite "except for" wording it is a significant finding

 

## Question 1:

B) Thyroid function

## Question 2:

E) Hypothyroidism

The coarse facies can divert you into picking one of the mucopolysaccharidoses such as Hurler, Hunter or Morquio syndrome. However the separated sutures, umbilical hernia and the fact that the child was born in a developing country should make for a clear diagnosis of hypothyroidism.

# Case 49

(see page 155 for Questions)

You are evaluating a 5-month-old infant with fine hair and a crusted rash that is concentrated around the face, hands and feet over the past 3 weeks. The infant has also not gained any weight over the past month and has been less energetic than usual and his stools have been loose, occasionally watery. He has been exclusively breast fed until 4 weeks ago when he was switched to iron based formula in anticipation of the mother returning to work.

Crusted rash around the face and extremities coupled with fine hair.

Coincides with the switch to formula

Weight loss, Loose stools, and lethargy

Timing coincides with onset of symptoms

## Question 1:

E) Acrodermatitis enteropathica

## Question 2:

E) Zinc supplements

## Question 3:

A) Hypogammaglobulinemia

The onset of symptoms coincides with the patient being weaned from breast milk to formula. It would be tempting to assume that this is due to cow milk allergy except the described rash is classic for zinc deficiency. In addition, poor weight gain, the thin hair and decreased energy are also consistent with zinc deficiency.

Breast milk contains an enzyme which enhances zinc absorption that is not present in cow based formula. Infants with *acrodermatitis enteropathica* have a defective transport enzyme resulting in poor GI absorption. Without the enhanced absorption afforded by breast milk *acrodermatitis enteropathica* typically manifests after an infant has been weaned.

As a secondary result of zinc deficiency, enzymes that are zinc dependent hypofunction, resulting in immunodeficiency including hypogammaglobulinemia.

Phrynoderma is seen in Vitamin A deficiency resulting in dry cracked skin. This is also known as *follicular hyperkeratosis.* Zinc supplementation results in resolution of the dermatological manifestations outlined in this vignette.

# Case 50

(see page 157 for Questions)

You are asked to consult on a 7-year-old girl because of development of fine pubic hair and hair on the inner thigh with breast budding.

By definition early pubertal development and abnormal

ANSWER REVEALED

True precocious puberty

Until recently she has been at the 50th percentile for weight and height but over the past 6 months has experienced an increase in height velocity.

Increased height velocity

She is taking no medications and has not been exposed to any drugs or toxins. She has not experienced any recent head trauma.

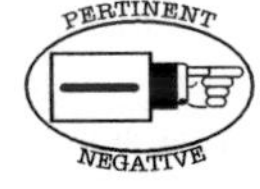


Trauma an unlikely explanation

She does not use any makeup.

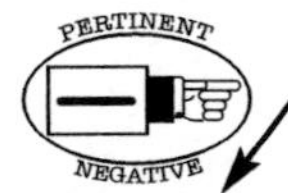


Exogenous exposure to estrogen unlikely

 

## Question 1:

E) Wrist x-ray

## Question 2:

C) Idiopathic early maturation of the hypothalamic pathway

## Question 3:

E) Ganciclovir and Foscarnet

The patient is female and younger than age 8 and has entered both thelarche and pubarche, which is by definition *precocious puberty.* They should note that the girl is Caucasian or else have a much younger age, however, on the boards since different ethnic groups can mature earlier within normal limits.

Children presenting with precocious puberty should initially be evaluated by bone age via x-ray of the wrist.

Advanced bone age would then require a GnRH stimulation test followed by head and/or abdominal CT depending on the results.

If the bone age is not advanced this would be more consistent with hypothyroidism. However the history would have to include other signs as well.

 

# Case 51

(see page 159 for Questions)

A 14-year-old girl presents with a 2-month history of pale patches on her skin, which is very concerning to her. On physical exam you note that the rash is limited to her chest and back and consists of hypopigmented scaling macules with several of them coalescing into patches with distinct borders. She has no history of atopic dermatitis or any other dermatological disorders.

Classic description of tinea versicolor

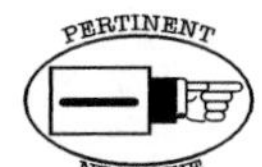


This rules out pityriasis alba which is associated with atopic dermatitis

## Question 1:

A) Tinea versicolor

## Question 2:

A) *Pityrosporum orbiculare*

## Question 3:

A) Topical antifungal agent

Tinea versicolor is caused by *Pityrosporum orbiculare*, which is a yeast. It causes hypopigmented scaly macules, which coalesce into distinct patches. (Note that this is the usual presentation. It can cause darker-colored macules in very fair skin.)

This can be distinguished from the following:

**Pityriasis Alba:** Occurs in patients with atopic dermatitis; also hypopigmented macules. However, in this case they appear on the face with *indistinct margins.*

**Vitiligo:** Lesions that are *completely depigmented*, not hypopigmented. They would also not be described as scaling.

The treatment of choice for Tinea versicolor is topical antifungal agents.

# Case 52

(see page 161 for Questions)

You are evaluating a 6-week-old infant with increasing levels of respiratory distress. On physical exam you note high-pitched inspiratory stridor that the parents confirm has been for the most part present since birth. There are no audible murmurs on physical examination and the child has otherwise been doing well.

Etiologies limited to those seen in 6-week-old infant

Inspiratory stridor, diseases limited to those that present with inspiratory stridor. Rules out etiologies that present with expiratory or biphasic stridor.

## Question 1:

B) Supraglottic mass

## Question 2:

A) Laryngomalacia

Foreign body aspiration, intrathoracic masses, and vascular compression all result in *expiratory stridor.*

Subglottic lesions often result in *biphasic* stridor.

In addition, foreign body aspiration would be unlikely in a 6-week-old since they are not mobile.

Inspiratory stridor (or biphasic stridor but more inspiratory than expiratory) would be consistent with a diagnosis of laryngomalacia, which would typically present in the newborn period and present from birth.

Tracheomalacia presents with expiratory stridor. A subglottic hemangioma would present with biphasic stridor. Epiglottitis and Laryngeal papillomatosis would not be appropriate diagnoses in this age group.

# Case 53

(see page 163 for Questions)

You are asked to evaluate a 15-year-old girl because of significant weight loss over the past 2.5 years when she has dropped from the 40th percentile for weight to the 10th percentile. The weight loss is very concerning to the parents and the girl. She is not taking any medications, has not experienced diarrhea or abdominal pain and has generally been asymptomatic except for occasional low-grade fevers, more than would be typical for her age. She also often feels full and bloated and tends to only have one or sometimes two meals a day. A stool sample is negative for O and P, negative for gross blood, and positive for

Self explanatory

Rules out an eating disorder

Suggests inflammatory bowel disease

Early satiation is consistent with Crohn's disease

## Question 1:

A) Crohn's Disease

## Question 2:

D) Nutritional rehabilitation

## Question 3:

D) Lower than expected adult height

Unexplained weight loss in the absence of abdominal pain can be a classic presentation of Crohn's disease, especially on the boards. The fact that the weight loss is of concern to the girl rules out an eating disorder as the explanation. In the absence of more significant diarrhea and abdominal symptoms ulcerative colitis is unlikely. The absence of systemic signs beyond the weight loss points against an occult malignancy. There are no indications of depression in this patient.

Up to one-third of patients with Crohn's disease will not reach their adult height potential and this is best countered with "nutritional rehabilitation" with nasogastric feedings if necessary.

# Case 54

(see page 165 for Questions)

Bilateral conjunctivitis 2 weeks post delivery

At the 2-week checkup you note that the infant has bilateral mucopurulent eye discharge with some swelling and erythema of the eyelids. You review the hospital record and note the baby was born by spontaneous vaginal delivery with apgars of 8 and 9 with a normal postnatal course. The baby was full term with a birth weight of 3200 grams. Silver nitrate drops were placed in both eyes. The baby has been otherwise feeding well and has regained birthweight.

Only provides protection against gonorrhea not chlamydia

## Question 1:

E) Chlamydia conjunctivitis

## Question 2:

C) Erythromycin ethylsuccinate orally

## Question 3:

C) Pneumonia

There is nothing in the history to suggest a risk for herpes therefore herpes keratitis is unlikely. Silver nitrate drops would protect against GC so there is little risk for permanent blindness if untreated. Dacryostenosis would most likely be unilateral, not bilateral.

Therefore given that silver nitrate drops protect against GC and not chlamydia and the timing of the bilateral discharge chlamydia is the most likely cause of the bilateral mucopurulent discharge.

The most important complication would be pneumonia, which can be prevented with oral erythromycin *not* topical ophthalmological ointment.

# Case 55

(see page 167 for Questions)

Newborn Rash

You are called to evaluate a rash on a 3-day-old infant by a frantic mother. On physical exam the child is afebrile, alert, and feeding well in the mother's arms. You note a rash on the face and chest which are erythematous macules measuring around 3 cm with a papule in the center.

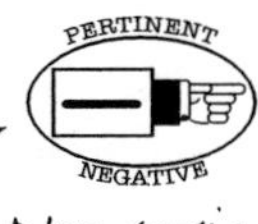


Non toxic

Classic description of erythema toxicum

The mother's prenatal history was unremarkable and the baby was born full term by normal spontaneous vaginal delivery. The mother does have a past history of genital herpes that has not been active in years.

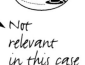

Not relevant in this case

## Question 1:

E) Erythema toxicum

## Question 2:

C) Wright Stain

## Question 3:

E) Reassurance

A newborn rash on the face and chest described as erythematous macules around 3 cm which have a papule in the center would be a classic description of erythema toxicum. Wright stain would reveal eosinophils and it is a benign rash of unknown etiology that requires no intervention.

# Case 56

(see page 169 for Questions)

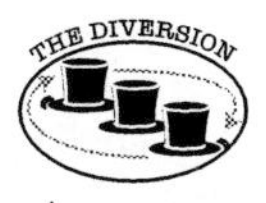


This is to mislead you into believing that that patient has rotavirus

You are taking care of an 18-month-old toddler who attends a day care center four days a week and presents with a several week history of watery diarrhea and moderate weight loss. On physical examination you note abdominal distension and low energy.

Prior to this point weight gain has been in the 75th percentile with normal growth and development.

Non-specific findings

Consistent with a diagnosis of giardiasis

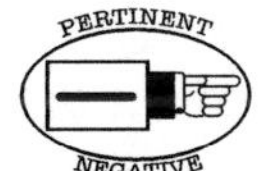


Rules out a chronic condition

## Question 1:

E) ELISA stool assay for Giardia

## Question 2:

A) Small bowel biopsy

## Question 3:

E) Metronidazole

In this question the diagnosis is not difficult. What you really need to clarify is:

- The most appropriate diagnostic step *in this patient*
- The most *sensitive* diagnostic step
- The best treatment

The correct diagnosis in this patient is giardiasis as evidence by the combination of watery diarrhea, abdominal distension, weight loss and fatigue. The diagnosis can be made in a variety of ways including

- Enzyme lined immunosorbent assay (ELISA) testing of the stools
- Entero-Test® string test
- Small bowel biopsy

While the small bowel biopsy would be the *most sensitive test* it would not be appropriate in *this patient.* The most appropriate test in this patient would be ELISA stool assay for Giardia. The best treatment would be metronidazole.

# Case 57

(see page 171 for Questions)

Acute Process

An 11-year-old boy presents with acute onset of swelling just in front of the ear at the jaw line. A school physical 3 months ago was within normal limits with no evidence of facial swelling or adenopathy.

The patient's immunization status is completely up to date.

Recent history of severe dehydration

Two weeks ago the patient did have a severe gastroenteritis and he was seen in the ER but the parents preferred oral rehydration rather than IV hydration as recommended by the pediatric ER attending.

Consistent with an acute infection

On physical examination you note marked right sided pre-auricular swelling with tender adenopathy and erythema of the overlying skin.

*(Continued on next page)*

Consistent with acute infection of Stensen duct

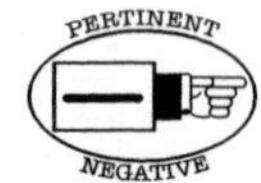


*(Continued from previous page)*

Examination of the oral cavity reveals a swollen red area on the lateral aspect of the floor below the tongue with malodorous discharge.

There is no evidence of dental caries. Tapping on the lower teeth does not result in any pain or discomfort.

Referral to Dentist or oral surgeon not indicated

## Question 1:

E) Treatment based on presentation

## Question 2:

C) Bacterial Parotitis

## Question 3:

E) Oral Cefazolin and Sour Lemon Candies

This patient is presenting with an acute process. Given that the child had a recent bout of severe dehydration and there is evidence of an acute infectious process involving Stensen's duct with malodorous discharge the most likely diagnosis is acute parotitis due to *Staph aureus*. Therefore no additional studies are necessary other than appropriate treatment.

In this, coverage can best be provided with cefazolin or amoxicillin/clavulanate. However, believe it or not the *best* treatment would include the addition of sour lemon candies, which serve as a *sialagogue*. Lemon candies are considered to be sialogogues since they would stimulate the salivary glands encouraging drainage. Perhaps even trying to pronounce the sialagogue would accomplish the same but this wasn't one of the choices.

We don't know what "Talking Tropical Parotitis" is. File that for your trip to the tropics for a conference of your choice upon successful completion of the exam.

# Case 58

(see page 175 for Questions)

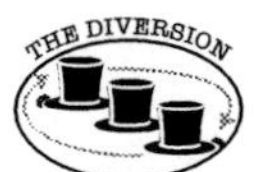


The initial story starts out benign leading you to believe that this is a simple story of constipation

You are treating a 5-year-old boy for constipation and intermittent abdominal pain, which has gotten worse over the past 3 months. Over the past weeks he has also been vomiting and not feeling well. The pain is intermittent with no set pattern. The parents can feel the stools and gas in the left lower abdomen just as you have on prior visits. You have given the parents instructions on increasing fiber in the diet, which has helped soften the stool, and decreased the severity of the constipation. You have also had to prescribe a stool softener. However the symptoms soon return as soon as the patient is taken off of stool softeners.

The boy has otherwise done fairly well

(Continued on next page)

This could be read as coincidental viral GE or a story of obstruction rather than the correct diagnosis.

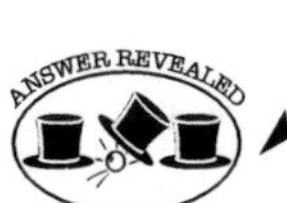


This is a very significant finding, which is camouflaged in wording which leads you to believe that the findings are consistent with the diagnosis of constipation. See elaboration below.

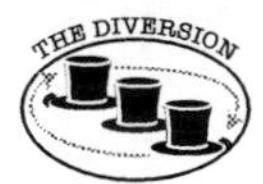


The fact that the constipation responded to dietary changes and treatment it is somewhat misleading but not that misleading since clearly the fact that it does not work is noted right away.

*(Continued from previous page)*

with no significant weight loss or fever. He is taking no medications at this time.

PHYSICAL EXAMINATION

Afebrile, HR 110, RR – 16

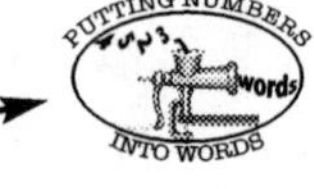


Blood pressure 119/ 82

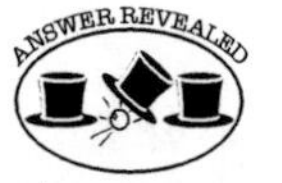


The physical findings clearly note a non tender abdominal mass which should make you think of a Wilms tumor

HEENT – PERRLA, TMs intact, and throat clear
Neck – Supple, no palpable lymph nodes

Lungs- Clear, no rhonchi, wheeze or rales

Abdomen – Positive normal bowel sounds, Left lower quadrant pain with radiation to the left flank.
In the left lower abdomen you palpate a firm non-tender mass. No guarding or rebound tenderness.

*(Continued on next page)*

(Continued from previous page)

Rectal exam – negative

LAB RESULTS

CBC –

WBC- 9.5 with a normal differential
H/H 12/34

Urinalysis

RBC- 7-10
WBC- 2
Negative Bacteria

PUTTING NUMBERS INTO WORDS

Microscopic hematuria

Abdominal x-ray – Non-obstructive pattern, hazy left sided mass that appears to be impacted stools

Noting the hazy pattern consistent with stool can certainly divert you to thinking that this is the correct diagnosis.
In a case like this you should also realize that the diagnosis is rarely so simple that the average person reading the question could get it right. I.e. X-ray shows stool therefore constipation is the correct diagnosis.

## Question 1:

D) Renal Ultrasound

## Question 2:

B) Abdominal CT with IV contrast

## Question 3:

A) Aniridia

The history in this vignette notes that the parents felt the same mass you the physician noted. However in this case you the physician had the wrong diagnosis. While there may have been stool in the colon, what you and the parents were palpating was a renal mass. *Frequently it is the parents who notice the abdominal mass while bathing the child or putting on their clothes and it is* *<u>they</u>* *who bring it to the attention of the physician.*

The *microscopic hematuria* should make you think of Wilms tumor. The hematuria and the back pain would be consistent with a renal stone but not the mass and the constipation.

The mild hypertension seen in this patient is consistent with Wilms tumor and constipation can be seen with the more common abdominal pain in patients with Wilms tumor.

Renal ultrasound would be the most appropriate initial study and once a mass is seen the CT with IV contrast would distinguish the mass as being intrarenal vs. extrarenal with the former being consistent with a diagnosis of Wilms tumor.

# Case 59

(see page 179 for Questions)

You are evaluating an 8 year old boy who according to the parents has been experiencing inappropriate flatulence and abdominal pain on weekend when he is out with friend in the park, particularly during the summer. He is very popular with a group that plays little league baseball and other than an ice cream party after his 2 games on Saturday and Sunday his diet is good. He has been diagnosed with atopic dermatitis which is kept under control with emollient cremes and he has not experienced any flare-ups in several years.

He drinks small amounts of milk occasionally and some dairy products with no difficulty although he tends to shy away from this.

Symptoms limited to weekends during the summer

THE DIVERSION

Red herring to lead you to the false belief that this is allergy related

Consumption of large amounts of ice cream

The atopic dermatitis is unrelated to the current presentation

**Small amounts** of dairy products have no impact

## Question 1:

C) Enzyme deficiency

## Question 2:

E) Lactase supplements

The patient experiencing flatulence, bloating and abdominal pain when consuming **large** amounts of dairy products (ice cream party) and no symptoms when consuming small amounts. This is consistent with lactose intolerance since patients who are lactose intolerant have some lactase activity allowing them to digest small amounts of dairy products.

If the patient had try milk allergy which is IgE mediated he could not even tolerate small amounts. The mention of atopic dermatitis is there to try to divert you away from the correct answer. However milk protein allergy would tend to make atopic dermatitis worse with dairy product ingestion and in this case the symptoms did not worsen helping to substantiate the diagnosis of lactose intolerance.

# Case 60

(see page 181 for Questions)

A 15-year-old girl has been experiencing recurrent headaches with increasing frequency. The headaches are bilateral and feel like a non-pulsating vise-grips tightening on both sides of her head. There has not been any recent head injury. She has not experienced any photophobia or nausea and she is able to carry out routine activities despite the pain.

Consistent with a tension headache

PERTINENT NEGATIVE

subdural hematoma unlikely

Her school performance has not changed despite it being difficult to concentrate because of the pain. She is very concerned about final exams coming up and has had a difficult time managing time.

Inconsistent with depression

*(Continued on next page)*

*(Continued from previous page)*

On physical examination the patient appears to be a bit anxious about her final exams. There is no papilledema; cranial nerves are within normal limits. Muscle tone and gait are within normal limits with 2+ deep tendon reflexes throughout.

Consistent with increased perception of stressful events, not necessarily clinical depression

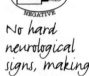

No hard neurological signs, making a space occupying lesion unlikely

## Question 1:

A) Referral for psychological counseling

## Question 2:

A) Tension headaches

## Question 3:

A) Analgesics and relaxation exercises

Headaches that are described as recurrent and bilateral that do not interfere with *everyday activity* are consistent with tension headaches. Patients with tension headaches tend to perceive stressful events with more anxiety. Therefore the most appropriate treatment would be psychological evaluation/counseling and analgesics.

The history and physical exam is inconsistent with pseudotumor cerebri or an explanation related to trauma such as a subdural hematoma. Unilateral pain which is throbbing accompanied by nausea and vomiting would be more consistent with a migraine headache.

Headaches could be a sign of depression however one would expect deterioration in school performance and other vegetative signs of depression such as increased or decreased sleep. It might have been tempting to pick benign exertional headaches but this is a diagnosis mostly reserved for adults and is a headache that is vascular in origin and more akin to migraine headaches.

 

# Case 61

(see page 185 for Questions)

You are evaluating an afebrile 13-month-old with a pruritic rash that started 2 weeks earlier and has been getting progressively worse. Although he has been fussy he has otherwise been asymptomatic. He was started on whole milk a week before his first birthday. He has never had any rash before. He lives with his mother, father, 5-year-old brother and 3-year-old sister; they have no rash or other concerning symptoms.

Non toxic

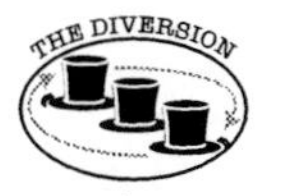


Red herring diversion to trick you into believing it is milk protein allergy causing the problem

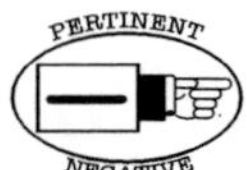


Makes a diagnosis of chronic illness such as milk allergy, or atopic dermatitis less likely

THE DIVERSION

scabies still possible even with asymptomatic siblings

On physical exam the rash is present on his trunk and extremities including the palms and soles of his feet. On the trunk you note even distributed red papules along with pustules on the soles of his feet.

Classic description of scabies

 

## Question 1:

C) Scabies infestation

## Question 2:

B) Permethrin 5 % for the patient and all family members

## Question 3:

C) Diphenhydramine

This patient has a classic presentation consistent with scabies. You cannot expect to be presented with a slam-dunk presentation of erythematous papules and burrows in the interdigital webs seen in older children or in adolescents where it can also be seen at the belt line and the flexure surfaces of the wrists and elbows.

When you are presented with a case of scabies they will often tell you that the rest of the family is asymptomatic to make a diagnosis of scabies trickier. Remember it can take up to 30 days from the time of infestation to the presentation of symptoms.

Even after successful treatment pruritic symptoms can continue. As long as new lesions do not appear this does not represent treatment failure. In this case antipruritic medication i.e. diphenhydramine is the only indicated treatment.

# Case 62

(see page 187 for Questions)

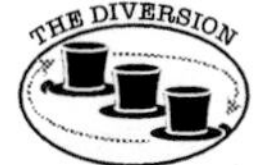


Clearly not the correct diagnosis

A 6-year-old boy is brought to your office by his frantic parents because they believe he is having a stroke. They returned 2 days earlier from a camping trip and the boy has otherwise been doing fine. He experienced no recent head trauma and his growth and development have been normal. The parents note that he has never even had a headache before.

Exposure to deer ticks good probability

Makes a tumor, stroke or migraine very unlikely

On physical examination the boy seems to be hypersensitive to sound and his right eyelid is opened. He is unable to keep it closed when you ask him to resist your attempts to open it. He has no trouble opening both eyes and his extraocular eye movements are intact. When you ask him to smile he

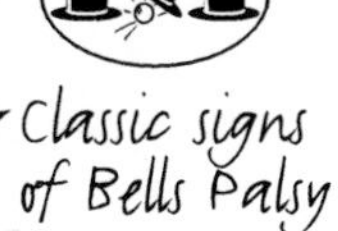


Classic signs of Bells Palsy

(Continued on next page)

*(Continued from previous page)*

can only smile on the left side.

His hearing and vision are completely normal.

He can't taste food on the anterior portion of his tongue and there is pain just below his right ear. The patient is experiencing no vertigo or dizziness.

ANSWER REVEALED

Classic signs of Bells Palsy

## Question 1:

E) Neuroborreliosis

## Question 2:

E) Lyme titers

## Question 3:

E) Excellent with full recovery within a few weeks

The patient in the vignette displays the classic signs of Bells Palsy, which is a palsy of the facial nerve. The cranial nerves are not involved and vision and hearing should not be impacted. However *hyperacusis* or high sensitivity to sound is a part of the scenario.

In an otherwise healthy child who just returned from a camping trip the most likely cause of the Bells Palsy would be Lyme disease. You didn't expect that to be one of the choices. The answer was called by the more formal name of Bells Palsy caused by Lyme disease, *neuroborreliosis.*

Therefore the most logical diagnostic step to take in this patient would be serum lyme titers. It is also one of the least invasive. The prognosis is excellent for the patient in the vignette with full recovery expected within a few weeks. You would, of course, treat isolated Lyme-related Bells Palsy with oral antibiotics – however, there is no evidence that they alter the clinical course of the facial paralysis.

 

# Case 63

*(see page 191 for Questions)*

An 8-year-old boy presents with a patchy distribution of hair loss over the past 8 weeks. On physical exam you note several area of hair loss with the exposed skin exhibiting a scaling appearance with black dots interspersed in some. The rest of the physical exam is unremarkable.

Classic description of tinea capitis

## Question 1:

D) Tinea capitis

## Question 2:

E) Potassium hydroxide preparation

## Question 3:

D) Oral antifungal

Tinea capitis is typically described as hair loss with the exposed skin exhibiting a scaling appearance with black dots interspersed in some. In addition it can be described as erythematous and boggy. The correct treatment is with an oral antifungal agent such as Griseofulvin. The best way to establish a diagnosis is by potassium chloride preparation, which will reveal the hyphae, which are diagnostic for the condition.

# Case 64

(see page 193 for Questions)

A 12-year-old boy has been gradually experiencing difficulty walking. On physical exam you note a hammer toe in the right foot with some atrophy of the muscles over the dorsal aspect of both feet as well as high arches bilaterally. The muscles of the legs appear to have moderate tone with what can best be described as a stork-like appearance. The muscles of the hands appear to be atrophied as well and look like "claw hands". Deep tendon reflexes are diminished in all 4 extremities. There is a negative Babinski sign.

Classic signs of Charcot-Marie-Tooth

Consistent with a peripheral neuropathy rather than an upper motor neuron problem

His growth and development have otherwise been normal. There is a family history for a muscle weakness but the parents are not clear on the details.

An inherited disorder

 

## Question 1:

A) EMG

## Question 2:

B) Charcot-Marie –Tooth Disease

Charcot-Marie-Tooth disease is a neuropathy that involves both *sensory* and *motor* dysfunction (motor much more pronounced). It typically is diagnosed between the age of 10 and twenty with distal motor weakness manifesting initially with weakness in the hands and feet.

BUZZ WORDS Watch out for buzz words such as "Stork like legs"," claw hand" and "high arched feet"

EITHER OR CHOICES Friedreich ataxia would present with high arches and ataxia, however the other signs are more consistent with Charcot-Marie- Tooth disease. In addition Friedreich ataxia also presents with cardiac disease and this would likely be included in the description.

---

**Reference:** Chance, PF, Pleasure D. Charcot –Marie –tooth syndrome. Arch Neurol. 1993;50:1180-1184

# Case 65

(see page 195 for Questions)

You are taking care of a 5-year-old boy in the 10th %ile for height. In addition you note bowing of the legs. His balanced diet has been documented by a nutritionist.

Short stature

Rickets

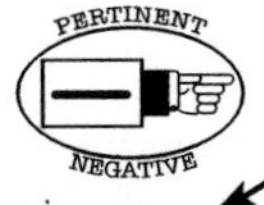


Dietary deficiency not a factor

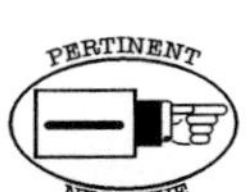


Laboratory findings include
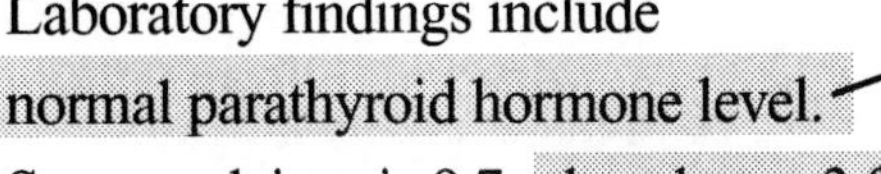
normal parathyroid hormone level. Serum calcium is 9.7, phosphorus 3.0, alkaline phosphatase of 790. Vitamin D 25 hydroxy is normal; Vitamin D 1, 25 dihydroxy is low.

Hypopara-thyroidism not a factor

Low serum phosphorus. Elevated Alkaline phosphatase

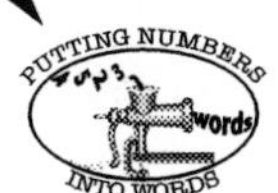


Low Vitamin D 1,25 (Activated Calcitriol) levels

 

## Question 1:

E) Familial hypophosphatemic rickets

## Question 2:

A) Calcitriol supplementation

The patient in this vignette has laboratory and clinical findings consistent with familial *hypopophosphatemia.*

They hypophosphatemia is due to phosphate loss in the kidneys and is associated with diminished conversion from Vitamin D 25, Hydroxy ( calcitriol) ➜ Vitamin D 1,25 Dihydroxy form (activated calcitriol) despite low phosphate levels which would ordinarily increase the conversion process.

Therefore in familial hypophosphatemia one would expect to see:

- Normal Vitamin D, 25 levels
- Low Vitamin D1,25
- Normal Serum Calcium
- Low Serum Phosphate
- Elevated alkaline phosphatase

Oral phosphate supplementation would be of no help. Calcitriol supplementation would be the treatment of choice.

You must be able to distinguish the very different and very confusing forms of rickets. Follow the bouncing hydroxylated D:

**Vitamin D deficiency** is due to; you guessed it, a nutritional deficiency of Vitamin D often coupled with inadequate sunlight exposure. Laboratory findings would include

- Low Serum phosphorus levels
- **Low Calcium**
- Elevated alkaline phosphatase
- **Hyperparathyroidism**
- **Vitamin D 25-hydroxy low (consistent with nutritional deficiency)**

### Vitamin D–independent rickets

Similar profile as Vitamin D deficiency except here the problem is with 1-hydroxylation at the kidney. Therefore:

- Vitamin D 25 hydroxy levels are normal
- Vitamin D 1,25 dihydroxy levels are so low you can't detect it (as opposed to low levels seen in this vignette)

### Vitamin D Dependent Rickets

Here there is end organ resistance to Vitamin D resulting in **very high levels of Vitamin D 1, 25 dihydroxy**

### Hypophosphatasia

The x-ray picture will be consistent with Rickets

## Renal Osteodystrophy

This is the result of **chronic renal failure** and *phosphate retention* and *decreased 1 hydroxylation* → *low calcitriol levels.* This results in:

- Low serum calcium
- **Elevated serum phosphate**
- Elevated parathyroid hormone (secondary hyperparathyroidism)
- Elevated alkaline phosphatase

# Case 66

(see page 197 for Questions)

Newborn Rash

You are called to evaluate a rash on a 3-day-old infant by a frantic mother. On physical exam the child is afebrile, alert, and feeding well in the mother's arms. You note a rash on the face and chest which is pustular with an erythematous base along with several hyperpigmented macules which include a collarette of scale.

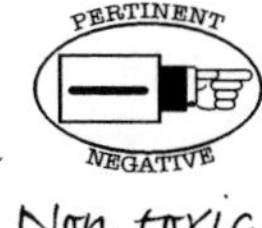


Non toxic

Classic description of transient neonatal pustular melanosis

The mother's prenatal history was unremarkable and the baby was born full term by normal spontaneous vaginal delivery. The mother does have a past history of genital herpes, which has not been active in years.

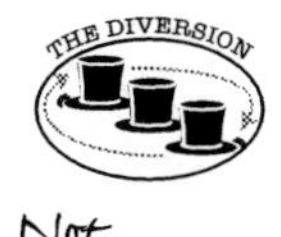


Not relevant in this case

## Question 1:

D) Transient neonatal pustular melanosis

## Question 2:

B) Gram Stain

## Question 3:

A newborn rash on the face and chest described as pustular with an erythematous base along with several hyperpigmented macules that include a collarette of scale would be a classic description of transient neonatal pustular melanosis. Gram stain would reveal polys and it is a benign rash of unknown etiology that requires no intervention

 

# Case 67

(see page 199 for Questions)

An 8-year-old boy presents with a patchy distribution of hair loss over the past 8 weeks. On physical exam you note one area of hair loss with hair of varying length.

Classic description of trichotillomania

There are no broken hairs noted and no erythema, scaling or black dots noted. The rest of the physical exam is unremarkable.

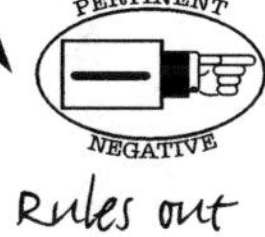


Rules out Tinea capitis

## Question 1:

B) Trichotillomania

## Question 2:

E) Stress reduction measures

Trichotillomania is due to repeated twirling or pulling hair usually in response to stress. *Hair loss of varying length* is a classic description. Therefore the best intervention is stress reduction measures since this is often the cause.

# Case 68

(see page 201 for Questions)

Multiple ingestion should be assumed automatically

A 16-year-old ingested a "fistful of pills" according to the group that brought her to the emergency room. She was non-responsive in the field and was intubated as a precaution. Your initial lab results include a toxicology screen positive for benzodiazepines and for acetaminophen. Liver function studies are pending. She was witnessed ingesting the pills 2 hours ago.

Confirms benzodiazepine ingestion.

Confirms acetaminophen ingestions

Timing is important. A level 2 hours from now would be the critical value to assess risk for hepatotoxicity

## Question 1:

A) Asymptomatic

## Question 2:

C) Administration of N-Acetylcysteine should be delayed based on an acetaminophen level in 2 hours.

## Question 3:

B) Administer Flumazenil immediately

Patients who have ingested a toxic dose of acetaminophen can be completely asymptomatic during the first 24 hours. After that period they would be at risk for hyperbilirubinemia, bleeding abnormalities, encephalopathy, and elevated LFT's and liver disease.

The most important lab value would be the acetaminophen level *4 hours post ingestion* since this is the best way of predicting the possibility of serious liver toxicity. Activated charcoal will not interfere with the absorption of N-Acetylcysteine if given in the recommended dosages. Therefore it should be given automatically to help decrease the absorption of additional acetaminophen.

Since this patient's tox screen was positive for benzodiazepines *flumazenil* as a benzodiazepine antagonist would be indicated regardless of anything having to do with the management of the acetaminophen toxicity.

# Case 69

(see page 205 for Questions)

You are evaluating a 4-year-old boy with a history of atopic dermatitis who presents with a severe rash on the extensor surface of his legs with a milder appearing rash on his arms and trunk. The rash can be best described as thin scales that have a pasted-on appearance with an elevated edge.

Condition associated with atopic derm, atopic derm cannot be the primary diagnosis, this would be too easy

Classic description and distribution of ichthyosis

The boy's father has a very similar appearing rash and there is a strong family history of asthma and allergies to environmental agents.

Inherited disorder

## Question 1:

E) Ichthyosis vulgaris

## Question 2:

E) Emollients

## Question 3:

B) Autosomal dominant

Ichthyosis vulgaris is an autosomal dominant disorder with scaly appearing skin that is often described as "pasted on". Up to 50% of children with ichthyosis vulgaris (ugly fish skin) also have atopic dermatitis, which is also associated with a family history of asthma and allergies to environmental agents. This is the diversion in the question but you should realize that they wouldn't blatantly give you the answer by naming the primary diagnosis by name in the history.

Ichthyosis vulgaris is *initially* treated with emollients.

 

# Case 70

(see page 207 for Questions)

A 3-year-old was found spitting out the contents of an opened bottle containing a liquid outdoor cleaner which is known to contain an acidic caustic substance. On physical examination the child is in no distress and you note that there are no lesions on the oral mucosa or pharynx.

Very simple, the assumption is the child ingested a known caustic substance

THE DIVERSION

This is noted to try to divert you into believing the child is in no danger and in no need of any intervention

 

## Question 1:

B) IV hydration

## Question 2:

B) Alkali ingestion is associated with a higher risk for perforation

## Question 3:

C) Endoscopy

Immediate treatment consists of IV fluids. The child should be NPO and activated charcoal, NG tubes and oral rehydration would be contraindicated.

Alkali burns tend to liquify tissue increasing the risk for perforation. Acid burns tend to result in coagulation necrosis decreasing the chance of perforation occurring.

The extent of tissue damage is unrelated to the volume ingested. Esophageal injury can be present even in the absence of any symptoms including dysphagia, chest pain, and drooling or oropharyngeal lesions.

Since the presence or absence of esophageal burns cannot be based on clinical symptoms all children suspected of ingesting caustic substances should undergo endoscopy regardless of clinical progress.

# Case 71

(see page 209 for Questions)

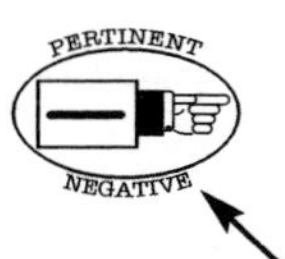


You are doing a school physical on a 15-year-old boy. He consistently gets A's and B's. His cardiac exam is normal although he does have a pectus excavatum, which the mother confided in you earlier that he is self-conscious about. He has previously participated and even excelled in sports but upon entering high school has withdrawn from all sports activity and is frequently out of breath while engaging in any activity at home or with close friends.

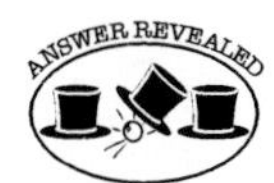


important hint that his self-consciousness is at the root of the problem

shortness of breath with no underlying physical explanation

## Question 1:

E) Lack of exercise

## Question 2:

E) Reassurance and encouragement to participate in sports

There is nothing in the history to suggest clinical depression in this child especially his good school performance. The normal cardiac exam points away from cardiac disease and there is nothing to suggest asthma or other pulmonary disease. Pectus excavatum does not result in compromised pulmonary function.

Most likely upon entering high school the boy is more self conscious about the deformity and as a result has withdrawn from participating in competitive sports and has fallen out of shape

Therefore reassurance and encouragement to participate in sports is the most appropriate treatment option in this patient.

 

# Case 72

(see page 211 for Questions)

You are called to the delivery room to evaluate a ten pound three ounce baby boy delivered vaginally. The delivery, as you could imagine, was difficult with marked shoulder dystocia.

High Risk for brachial plexus injury

The nurses are concerned because the infant is not moving his right arm well. You note that the baby is maintaining his upper arm in an internally rotated position with the shoulder adducted close to the body with his lower arm pronated and wrist flexed.

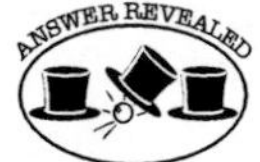


This is the classic waiter's tip presentation of Erb Palsy

## Question 1:

B) Erb Palsy

## Question 2:

A) Anhidrosis on the right side

## Question 3:

B) Some improvement within one month

The combination of shoulder dystocia and the classic waiter's tip presentation of Erb Palsy should make this a relatively easy series of questions to answer, especially the one calling for the correct diagnosis.

Erb palsy is associated with *Horner's Syndrome* and *diaphragmatic paralysis.* Of course Horner's syndrome is not listed as one of the associations. To answer this question correctly you would have to know that Horner's syndrome includes among other things *miosis* and *anhidrosis*[1] *of the ipsilateral side* which in this case is the right side.

[1] Which means "lack of sweating" which will hopefully describe you on the exam day since you are preparing meticulously

# Case 73

(see page 213 for Questions)

A 15-year-old boy is brought to your office. He appears to be healthy and is active in several sports. He is alarmed because he woke up in the morning and noticed that his eyes were yellow. However when he returns from school in the afternoon his eyes are white again. However this has been going on for over a week and he is concerned.

Jaundice worse in the morning

He does not drink any alcohol or take drugs, he is not sexually active and has no body piercing or tattoos. His physical exam is unremarkable including a soft abdomen with no guarding, rebound or hepatosplenomegaly. His bilirubin is 2.3 over 0.1 and his liver function tests are negative. All of his immunizations are up to date including the hepatitis B series which he received at birth.

Very low risk for hepatitis A through C

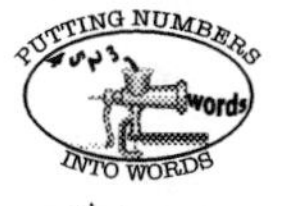


Mild unconjugated hyperbilirubinemia with normal LFT's

Especially low risk for hepatitis B

 

## Question 1:

D) Gilbert syndrome

## Question 2:

E) No further evaluation is necessary

## Question 3:

E) Occasional episodes of mild jaundice otherwise excellent

Mild jaundice which is worse in the morning in an otherwise healthy teenager is classic of Gilbert Syndrome which is a genetic disorder that is worse with fasting and therefore typically worse in the morning when most people cannot sleep and eat at the same time.

It is a diagnosis made on history and physical especially when there is no evidence of liver disease based on laboratory and physical findings. Therefore no additional testing is necessary.

Other than similar relatively benign episodes in the future the prognosis is excellent.

# Case 74

(see page 215 for Questions)

An 8-year-old boy is new to your practice. The mother heard about your stellar reputation and excellent taste in starchy white coats and tacky novelty ties. Her concern is over her son's repeated sinus infections with no explanations provided by the previous pediatrician whose lack of taste in ties rivals and usually exceeds yours. His old chart arrives on your desk with a thud that knocks your CD collection off the hanging plastic CD holder.

It is not clear if these are actual sinus infections

You note that in the past 3 years he has had 6 sinus infections and a few ear infections. Height and weight are in the 75th percentile for age and his development is within normal limits.

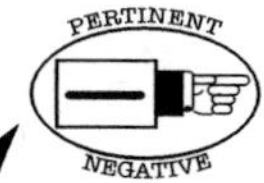


 

## Question 1:

E) Chronic allergic rhinitis

## Question 2:

E) Trial of intranasal steroids

Remember if a patient on the boards is presenting with an undiagnosed chronic illness they will more likely set it up as a patient presenting from a developing country and not a "developing cross town pediatric rival". In addition, the patient's normal growth and development would not be consistent with an undiagnosed immunodeficiency. The most likely explanation for the patient's history is chronic allergic rhinitis.

# Case 75

(see page 217 for Questions)

You are evaluating a 13-year-old boy for severe chest pain and shortness of breath. He is enrolled in a special education program because according to the parents "he is slow".

*Symptoms which should be taken seriously*

*Implies congnitive impairment which rules out Marfan Syndrome*

On physical examination he is thin for his age with scoliosis.

Ophthalmological examination reveals posterior displaced lenses.

*Classic for homocystinuria, distinguishing it from Marfan syndrome which presents with anterior lens displacement*

There is a normal S1 S2 with no murmurs or gallops noted. Capillary refill is less than 2 seconds.

*Cardiac function is normal*

He is afebrile with a pulse of 92 and respiratory rate of 64. Portable chest x-ray is negative.

PUTTING NUMBERS INTO WORDS

*Tachypneic*

## Question 1:

E) Chest CT

## Question 2:

A) Pulmonary embolus

## Question 3:

D) Homocystinuria

The presentation of a patient with shortness of breath, severe chest pain, and tachypnea should be enough to establish a working diagnosis of pulmonary embolus and the necessity of a chest CT scan. You are now 2/3 of the way to answering all the questions correctly.

The thin body should narrow you down to 3 choices, Marfan syndrome, Klinefelter and Homocystinuria. However there are no other features of Klinefelter's in this patient. In addition, this patient is in special education because he is "slow" implying cognitive impairment, which is not a feature of Marfan syndrome (which presents with *anterior* not posterior lens displacement). Therefore the correct underlying diagnosis is homocystinuria.

# Case 76

(see page 219 for Questions)

At the 2-week followup visit you notice that the neonate is slightly icteric.

*Jaundiced at 2 weeks post natal*

You review the neonatal record and discover that he had mild physiological jaundice which resolved after 5 days.

*Physiologic jaundice resolved*

He has already surpassed his birth weight, is breast-feeding well and producing loose mustard colored stools on a regular basis.

*Thriving*

On physical examination he is icteric down to the thighs with symmetrical muscle tone and strength and is alert and responsive. Abdomen is soft, non-tender with no hepatosplenomegaly.

*Icteric*

PERTINENT NEGATIVE

His total and direct bilirubin is 18/ 0.5

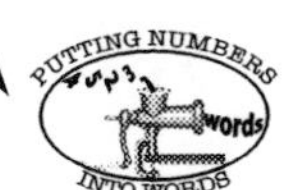


*Unconjugated hyperbilirubinemia*

## Question 1:

D) Breast milk jaundice

## Question 2:

D) Discontinue breastfeeding for 48 hours then resume

## Question 3:

E) Less than 2%

It is important to distinguish jaundice associated with breastfeeding from *breastfeeding jaundice.*

**Jaundice associated with breastfeeding** is essentially physiologic jaundice with higher bilirubin levels than in non-breast-fed neonates. In this case breastfeeding is *not* discontinued, it should if anything be increased.

**Breast-milk jaundice** occurs later around 2 weeks of age. In this case all that is needed is to interrupt breastfeeding for 48 hours. Breast milk jaundice occurs in around 2% of breast-fed infants.

There is no evidence of CMV or galactosemia in this infant.

# Case 77

(see page 221 for Questions)

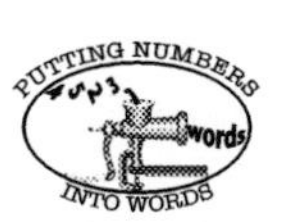


Actually we are turning words into numbers. This is roughly 53 mg/kg ingested

A 3-year-old toddler was found with an opened bottle of over–the-counter 200 mg ibuprofen tablets with half chewed tablets in his mouth. The ingestion occurred roughly 4 hours ago. The child weighs 15 kg and there were twenty pills in the bottle and sixteen are left. On physical examination the child is comfortable eating ice cream and remains playful. Vital signs are stable.

4 hours post ingestion

stable 4 hours post ingestion

 

## Question 1:

E) Observation only

## Question 2:

E) Observation only

## Question 3:

B) Acute respiratory distress syndrome

It is important to note that with ibuprofen ingestion, just like acetaminophen ingestion, 4 hours post ingestion is the important time frame.

Here, however, you do not need to draw levels of ibuprofen, however if one of the choices was to draw a salicylate and acetaminophen level this would be correct since you need to make sure there were not co-ingestions.

Children who ingest less than 100 mg/kg can be observed at home, so in this scenario with less than 100mg/kg ingested and with a clinically stable child nothing more than observation is needed.

At levels of 200-400 mg/kg ingested there is an increased risk for side effects so activated charcoal would be indicated. Levels greater than 400 would require serious observation as an inpatient.

Mild side effects include mostly GI, nausea, and vomiting, abdominal pain. Diplopia and headache can also occur. Serious side effects, which are quite rare, would include seizures, apnea and even bradycardia. Acute respiratory distress syndrome would not even be a rare side effect of ibuprofen ingestion.

# Case 78

(see page 223 for Questions)

You are evaluating a 6-year-old girl who is experiencing abdominal pain without any nausea or diarrhea. In addition she has been experiencing urinary frequency and diurnal enuresis with no dysuria. On physical exam there is left lower quadrant tenderness with no guarding or rebound with increased bowel sounds.

PERTINENT NEGATIVE

Points away from an acute abdomen

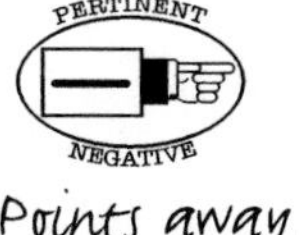


Points away from a UTI

Consistent with constipation

## Question 1:

A) Plain abdominal film

## Question 2:

B) Encopresis

## Question 3:

B) Increase dietary fiber

Patients with chronic constipation or encopresis can present with diurnal urinary incontinence. In this case a workup for constipation beginning with a plain abdominal film would be appropriate and treatment would consist of cleanout, increased dietary fiber and behavioral considerations.

# Case 79

(see page 225 for Questions)

Otalgia

An 8-year-old boy presents with severe right-sided ear pain of one week's duration that has interfered with his sleep. He plays goalie for his ice hockey team on a regular basis and wears protective equipment and does not recall sustaining any significant trauma. The pain radiates to the chin and neck and improves somewhat with ibuprofen but never fully.

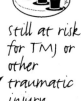

Still at risk for TMJ or other traumatic injury

He has had no sore throat symptoms, nasal discharge, dysphagia, or discharge from the ear. On physical examination there is no tenderness on movement of the outer ear, there is a clear view of the tympanic membrane with no inflammation and a positive light reflex with all landmarks visible. The throat is clear with no erythema or exudate noted. No oral lesions noted.

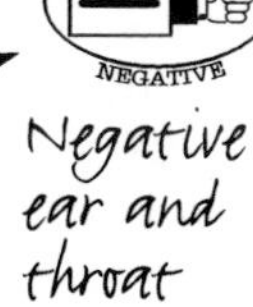


Negative ear and throat exam

## Question 1:

D) Temporomandibular joint syndrome

## Question 2:

E) Dental Workup

The patient in this vignette is presenting with ear pain or otalgia with a negative ear and throat exam. They note that he plays hockey as a goalie and despite the denial of any trauma and the use of protective equipment it is possible to sustain an injury and not know about it. In particular, if he is not wearing a protective mouth guard he could have sustained an injury to his TMJ joint and or be clenching his teeth during the game. In addition, even without this history children can be "teeth grinders" and have TMJ syndrome.

The response to ibuprofen is further evidence that joint inflammation could be the cause of the problem.

# Case 80

(see page 227 for Questions)

You are evaluating a 14-year-old basketball player who twisted his ankle coming down for a rebound. He arrived in your office bearing weight with a significant limp. On physical examination you note pain and swelling over the lateral ankle with both passive and active movement. You do not see any evidence of a fracture on x-ray.

Can be pre-pubescent and at risk for growth plate injury = Salter Harris I fracture

THE DIVERSION

Bearing weight does not rule out a severe sprain or a Salter Harris I fracture

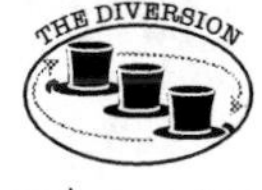


Salter Harris I fractures can easily be missed on x-ray

## Question 1:

C) Splint with no weight bearing

## Question 2:

A) Salter Harris 1 Fracture

## Question 3:

E) Heat

In this vignette it is important to note that pain over the lateral ankle can be indicative of a Salter Harris 1 fracture. This is because the weakest link in the ankle chain is the growth plate, not the ligaments. A Salter Harris 1 fracture can be invisible on x-ray or easily missed because it is only a minor separation of the growth plate. However it needs to be splinted like any fracture and therefore it is important to splint the injury with no weight bearing.

Because it can so easily be missed a Salter Harris fracture is the most concerning fracture.

The immediate management is RICE, rest, ice, compression and elevation. Heat is not part of the word RICE.

 

# Case 81

*(see page 229 for Questions)*

A 6-month-old child presents with a pruritic rash. On physical exam you note scaling of the scalp and the flexural folds of the extremities. There is also a greasy appearance of the scalp lesions. There is no evidence of diaper rash. There is no rash on other family members.

Classic description of seborrhea

 

## Question 1:

D) Seborrhea

## Question 2:

D) Application of baby oil

This vignette is a classic description of an infant with seborrhea or cradle cap. The only treatment is application of baby oil and use of a mild infant shampoo.

# Case 82

(see page 231 for Questions)

You are evaluating a 15-year-old who is presenting with a sore throat so painful it is difficult to swallow. He has a temperature of 102.4 and you note marked erythema of his pharynx with no exudate and his right tonsil is more swollen than the left, with the uvula shifter to the left. He has no respiratory stridor but is in a great deal of pain.

PERTINENT NEGATIVE

No evidence of viral croup

**Unilateral tonsillar swelling**, diagnostic for peritonsillar abscess

His immunizations are up to date and he has been otherwise doing well.

Epiglottitis unlikely

 

## Question 1:

B) Peritonsillar abscess

## Question 2:

C) Incision and drainage

## Question 3:

E) IV antibiotic coverage for Group A streptococcus and anaerobes

This patient is presenting with classic signs of peritonsillar abscess. There is no time to waste with diagnostic testing and although one could argue for intubation to protect the airway, incision and drainage of the abscess would alleviate the pain, reduce the risk for airway obstruction dramatically and also allow for culture.

Until culture results are back the most appropriate step to take would be IV antibiotics providing coverage for Group A strep and anaerobes.

# Case 83

*(see page 233 for Questions)*

You are evaluating a 2-year-old with "chronic otitis externa" with discharge. Despite a course of ofloxacin otic and appropriate oral antibiotics the otorrhea continues. There is no known history of barotrauma and the parents do not recall anything being placed in the ear. The child is afebrile with normal growth and developmental milestones. On physical examination it is difficult to visualize the tympanic membrane because of cerumen and other debris. There is no pain on manipulation of the outer ear.

Quotations, presumed but not confirmed diagnosis

Does NOT rule out foreign body or barotrauma

Failed topical and oral antibiotic course

Rules out any chronic hearing deficit or related problems

Removal of cerumen is a priority

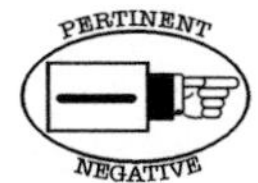


Rules out otitis externa

## Question 1:

E) Foreign body

## Question 2:

D) Gentle irrigation of the ear

The combination of otorrhea and no response to topical and oral antibiotics in a 2-year-old raises the suspicions for a foreign body in the ear. With the TM obstructed by cerumen its removal is a priority and the best way to do this at this point would be gentle irrigation. This may, in addition to removing the cerumen, dislodge the foreign body as well.

# Case 84

(see page 235 for Questions)

PERTINENT NEGATIVE

You are evaluating a 2-year-old toddler who has been experiencing increasing diarrhea which continues despite several attempts to modify the child's diet. With the exception of the first stool of the day, the stools are loose and malodorous with visible food particles noted during diaper changes. Growth and development are within normal limits for all parameters. His appetite is normal for age.

Unlikely to be celiac sprue, milk allergy

Formed first stool of the day is classic of non-specific diarrhea in toddlers.

Too non-specific to help

Suggests a disorder that is short-lived

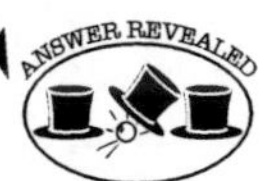


Suggests increased GI motility, not mal-absorption

## Question 1:

A) Altered gastrointestinal motility

## Question 2:

B) Increase fat content to above 4-6 g/kg/day

The clinical vignette is classic for chronic *non-specific diarrhea* or toddlers diarrhea. This is considered to be a variation of irritable bowel syndrome seen in adults and is due to increased GI motility, which is caused by increased sorbitol in the diet, increased carbohydrates or insufficient fat content in diet.

The presence of formed food in the stool should not lead you to mistakenly believe that a malabsorption syndrome is the cause. There is nothing in the history to suggest a diagnosis of giardiasis.

With giardiasis you would expect to also see *fatigue, abdominal distension,* and *weight loss.*

Therefore the correct management is to increase fat content to above 4-6g/kg.

 

# Case 85

*(see page 237 for Questions)*

A 13-month-old child presents with a pruritic rash that has been recurring since the age of 9 months. On physical exam you note large areas of hypopigmentation on the upper extremities, which are scaly and chapped. There is marked scaling on the flexure surfaces. There is no evidence of diaper rash. There is no rash on other family members. Other than asthma the family history is negative.

Chronic problem

Classic description and distribution of atopic dermatitis

PERTINENT NEGATIVE

Very significant, family history of asthma is associated with atopic dermatitis

 

## Question 1:

A) Atopic dermatitis

## Question 2:

A) Emollients and hydrocortisone 1%

The description and distribution of the rash is classic for atopic dermatitis. Hypopigmentation is a classic sign of atopic dermatitis. The most important treatment is skin emollients and hydrocortisone cream.

Sparing of the diaper area is a classic sign and clue they will give you indicating that atopic dermatitis is the correct diagnosis.

# Case 86

(see page 239 for Questions)

You are evaluating a full term newborn who is tachypneic with audible rales. He was born via spontaneous vaginal delivery with no complications. On physical examination pulses to both the arms and legs are diminished and, other than an audible gallop, there are no cardiac murmurs. On cardiac echo systolic ejection fraction is normal and there is no evidence of congenital heart disease. Chest x-ray shows increased vascular markings.

*Congenital problem*

*Suggests increased pulmonary blood flow and congestion*

*Decreased circulation to upper and lower extremities*

*Left heart function is normal*

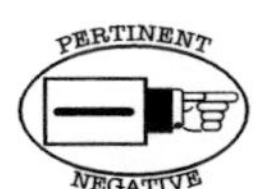


*No congenital cardiac disease*

## Question 1:

C) Intracranial arteriovenous malformation

## Question 2:

B) Diminished left ventricular function

When approaching a vignette that is potentially cardiac in etiology you want to go about it systematically and establish important facts. In this vignette the important facts that are laid out in the question itself are as follows:

1) Congenital
2) Pulmonary blood flow is increased
3) Circulation below the carotids is diminished.
4) The heart is normal
5) Left heart function is normal

Therefore you can conclude that there is a problem outside the heart that is decreasing blood flow to the lower part of the body and increasing it to the lungs.

What would "steal" blood from arterial circulation and send it to the lungs depriving the lower part of the body, but without anomalies on echo? The only logical answer would be an intracranial arteriovenous malformation.

Children with an AV malformation have the following features

- Shunting of systemic arterial blood directly to venous circulation *bypassing capillary beds*
- This increases pulmonary blood flow ➔ pulmonary congestion and *tachypnea*

 

- *L sided pre-load increases* eventually leading to *congestive heart failure*

Despite this the cardiac echo will be normal. If the AV shunt is cerebral there will be *decreased pulses in the extremities.* Arteriovenous malformations can also occur in the liver but this would not result in decreased pulses in the extremities as is the case in this vignette.

Initially left ventricular function should be normal eventually leading to diminished left ventricular function if untreated.

# Case 87

(see page 241 for Questions)

You are caring for a 7-year-old boy who has moved to your area with his family. You review his old chart and notice that he has had 3 episodes of lobar pneumonia requiring hospitalization for several days. In addition he has had one episode of documented osteomyelitis requiring hospitalization. He is afebrile with clear lungs and normal cardiac exam with no murmurs. There are several shoddy submandibular lymph nodes.

Serious infections not normal variations

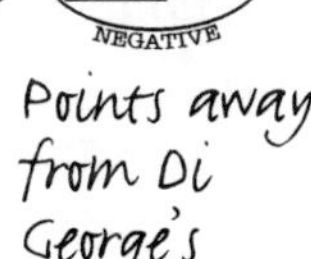


Points away from Di George's syndrome

Rules out X-linked agammaglobinemia

His CBC shows a WBC of 12.5 with a normal differential, hematocrit is 32, hemoglobin 11.5 and an MCV of 95. Platelet count is 175K.

Normocytic anemia

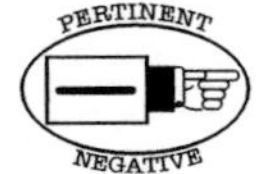


Normal platelet count rules out Wiskott Aldrich

## Question 1:

C) Chronic granulomatous disease

## Question 2:

E) Hepatosplenomegaly

## Question 3:

E) Mutation in X- chromosome

This is a vignette requiring you to note that the patient does have a defect placing him at risk for more serious infections than usual. By carefully reviewing the history, physical and labs you can eliminate all the choices except for the correct one.

The normal platelet count rules out Wiskott Aldrich, the presence of lymph nodes rules out agammaglobulinemia and the absence of cardiac symptoms essentially rules out Di George's since they would have to present Di George are with some classical signs.

The patient has anemia of chronic illness.

# Case 88

(see page 243 for Questions)

You are evaluating a 6-year-old boy who has been limping on his left leg for 4 weeks. His history is negative except for a minor fall while playing basketball around the time the limp started.

Onset with minor injury out of proportion with symptoms

He has had no recent viral illnesses and there is no significant past medical history.

PERTINENT NEGATIVE

Makes Lyme, JRA and septic arthritis unlikely

On physical exam he is afebrile with some pain over the inguinal area increased with abduction of the leg, which is limited.

Classic presentation of Legg Calve Perthes disease

## Question 1:

E) Frog left AP x-ray of the pelvis

## Question 2:

E) Legg Calve Perthes disease

Legg Calve Perthes disease often presents with limping after a minor trauma out of proportion with the symptoms. It can also present with a painless limp. Pain over the inguinal area is another classic symptom.

The best way to establish the diagnosis is with standard AP, frog leg x-ray of the pelvis.

# Case 89

(see page 245 for Questions)

You are evaluating a 16-year-old male in the emergency department for chest pain. She describes the pain as being constant and keeping her up at night. Ibuprofen has been of no help–the pain is much worse when he is lying down and he must lie down at an angle in order to sleep. He does much better sitting or standing up and has experienced no shortness of breath. His EKG was normal and his cardiac echo exam showed no compromise in cardiac function.

Constant chest pain resistant to ibuprofen rules out costochondritis

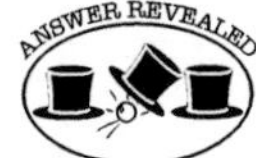


Chest pain worse in the supine position is typical of pericarditis

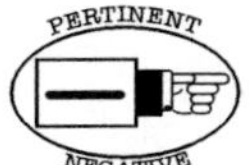


Rules out myocarditis

 

## Question 1:

C) Pericarditis

## Question 2:

E) Pericardial tamponade

## Question 3:

A) Adenovirus

This patient is experiencing unrelenting chest pain which does not respond to ibuprofen and is worse while lying down.

Pericarditis is often viral in origin including adenovirus as well as Coxsackie virus. Cardiac tamponade would be a complication of pericarditis if it leads to a pericardial effusion severe enough to interfere with cardiac function.

# Case 90

(see page 247 for Questions)

High risk for undiagnosed chronic illness or disease rarely seen in US due to immunization

You are evaluating an 18-month-old boy who immigrated from Guatemala two months ago. He presents with a fever of 103.5 F, with a severe cough, inflammation of the nares and rhinorrhea. His eyes are red and inflamed as well. In addition you note a macular rash concentrated behind his ears as well as his face and trunk.

Cough, Coryza and Conjunctivitis, the 3 C's of Measles

Typical rash seen in measles

 

## Question 1:

B) Rubeola

## Question 2:

A) Vitamin A

This patient presents with the 3 C's of Measles and is at high risk for measles because of his recent immigration from Guatemala. The rash is also typical of measles infection.

The morbidity and mortality of measles infection can be reduced with oral vitamin A supplementation.

# Case 91

*(see page 249 for Questions)*

You are evaluating a 17-year-old female for a routine physical examination. While taking the history she confirms that she has been sexually active and prefers not to tell her parents. She last had sexual relations 6 weeks ago and once before that with a different partner. She is pretty sure that both boys used condoms. Her last menstrual period was 2 weeks ago. She is not experiencing any dysuria, dysmenorrhea, or abdominal pain. Her urine HCG is negative.

*Better to assume that condoms were not used*

THE DIVERSION

*Asymptomatic for PID but still needs screening*

*Pregnancy ruled out*

## Question 1:

E) Urine DNA amplification test for Gonorrhea and Chlamydia

## Question 2:

C) American Cancer Society recommendations include delay of Pap screening until 3 years after onset of sexual activity

Even though this patient is asymptomatic for PID she is still at risk because it is never clear if appropriate protection was used. With the availability of urine DNA amplification it would be appropriate to screen an asymptomatic sexually active adolescent for Chlamydia and Gonorrhea since a more invasive pelvic can be avoided.

Regarding the Pap smear, in teenagers high-grade squamous intraepithelial lesions are rare and low-grade lesions frequently regress spontaneously. Therefore the American Cancer Society recommends postponing the Pap smear until 3 years after the onset of sexual activity (or age 21, whichever comes first). This is done with a pelvic examination since there is no DNA amplification urine screen to detect cervical cancer.

It will be interesting to see how things change with the new HPV or cervical cancer vaccine, which was just approved at time of printing.

# Case 92

(see page 251 for Questions)

You are evaluating a newborn male. The mother has been breastfeeding the baby every 3 hours as needed. The mother is very concerned because the baby has not passed a stool in 5 days. On physical examination of the baby there are no significant findings and the abdomen is soft and non-tender.

Normal breastfeeding pattern

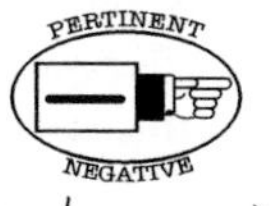


Rules out obstruction

The baby was full-term and delivered by normal spontaneous vaginal delivery with no complications. Apgars were 9 at one minute and five minutes. The baby has lost 4% of his birthweight and he passed a meconium stool within 24 hours.

PUTTING NUMBERS INTO WORDS

Well within normal limits

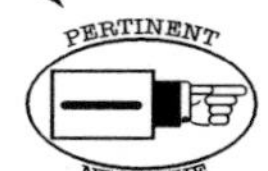


Rules out anal atresia and stenosis

## Question 1:

E) Reassurance

## Question 2:

B) Low initial volume of breast milk

This is a case where all that is needed is reassurance. The baby is breastfeeding normally, is not dehydrated and shows no signs of any disorder that would be concerning. The decreased stool is due to low initial breast milk volume, which will resolve as more breast-milk is produced as part of the process.

 

# Case 93

(see page 253 for Questions)

Hot weather

A 16-year-old girl was taking a walk with her sister along the beach during August. Earlier in the day she received a text message from her boyfriend informing her that he was out of state and ending their relationship. While they were walking the girl felt light-headed and quickly sat down and subsequently passed out in her sister's arms. Just before passing out, her face turned red and she was perspiring. The episode lasted less than a minute and you have been asked to evaluate her as a precaution. Except for nausea she has remained asymptomatic since the episode. She was recently started on a tricyclic antidepressant.

Emotional distress

Syncope preceded by diaphoreses and facial flushing

Increased risk for heat exhaustion

PUTTING NUMBERS INTO WORDS

Vital signs stable

Her blood pressure was 119/79 standing and sitting with a pulse rate of 72. She is afebrile. Her EKG showed normal sinus rhythm with no abnormalities noted.

No evidence of long QT syndrome

 

## Question 1:

D) Heat exhaustion

## Question 2:

C) She should remain indoors drinking copious amount of fluids

The girl in the vignette was walking on a hot summer day and was in emotional distress. In addition she was taking tricyclic antidepressants which place her at high risk for heat exhaustion. In such cases syncope would be preceded by facial flushing and diaphoreses.

There was no evidence of hyperventilation and there is enough physiological explanation for her syncope to make conversion disorder unlikely.

Heatstroke is a much more serious event which would present with *high temperature* and *altered state of consciousness.* Heatstroke would be a medical emergency requiring, among other things, IV fluids. Heat exhaustion on the other hand would only mandate that the patient go indoors and drink copious amount of fluids.

 

# Case 94

(see page 255 for Questions)

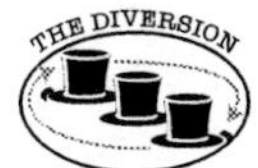


Attempt to mislead to a diagnosis of an eating disorder.

During a routine physical examination a 16-year-old teenager notes that she is very concerned about being overweight.

On physical examination her weight is above the 95th percentile and her heights are in the 92nd percentile for her age. Her neck is supple and there are no palpable masses noted. The rest of her physical examination is unremarkable.

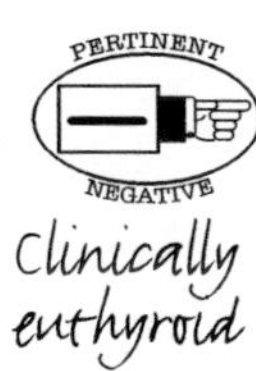


Laboratory studies include a:

CBC 10.5 with a Hematocrit of 39 and hemoglobin 12.5 with normal differential. Her serum sodium is 139, potassium 4.0, Chloride of 107, Bicarb 24, Glucose 90, Bun 25, creatinine 0.8.

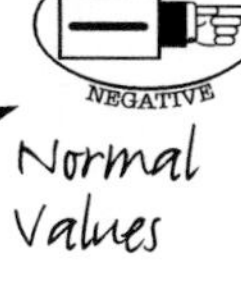


(Continued on next page)

(Continued from previous page)

Serum thyroxine level is low but Free T4 levels and TSH are both normal. $T_3$ resin uptake is elevated.

 

## Question 1:

D) Thyroid-binding globulin deficiency

## Question 2:

D) Serum thyroid binding globulin levels

Patients with thyroid-binding globulin deficiency are clinically "euthyroid" and have normal free T4 levels. However, since serum thyroxine includes both bound and unbound thyroxine, this will be low since it factors in bound T4. With fewer binding sites available on thyroid globulin, the $T_3$ resin uptake will be increased.

Since the patient's concern over her weight is legitimate she does not have anorexia nervosa or any other eating disorder.

The diagnosis that makes the most sense is thyroid binding globulin deficiency and measuring serum thyroid binding globulin levels is the best way to confirm this

# Case 95

(see page 259 for Questions)

You are evaluating a 3-year-old girl in the emergency room who presents with wheezing and respiratory distress with no improvement with 2 albuterol aerosols in the field and one upon arrival in the ED. She is lethargic and diaphoretic with increased salivation. Her eyes are miotic with pupils equal and reactive to light. The wheezing continues but she is able to breathe on her own. Her cardiac exam in normal and you note increased bowel sounds. Just prior to this she was playing in her grandfather's garden.

Poor response to albuterol aerosol consistent with a toxic exposure

Intubation not indicated

Increased risk for exposure to pesticides

ANSWER REVEALED

Consistent with organo-phosphate exposure

 

## Question 1:

B) Organophosphate toxicity

## Question 2:

E) Remove clothing and bathe

## Question 3:

D) IV Atropine

The patient in this vignette was playing in her grandfather's garden, which makes exposure to organophosphate containing pesticides very likely. In addition. this patient is presenting with classic signs of organophosphate toxicity including, sweating, tearing, salivation and GI stimulation.

Wheezing that does not respond to albuterol aerosols is another classic finding in organophosphate toxicity.

Since organophosphates can be absorbed through the skin and lungs and not just orally, the most appropriate step would be to undress and bathe (the patient, of course).

Once stabilized, atropine would be the appropriate antidote to use initially in organophosphate toxicity.

# Case 96

(see page 261 for Questions)

You are evaluating a 12-year-old girl who is just getting over an upper respiratory tract infection. The parents note that the cold only lasted 3 days because of the homemade tea she was given. Unfortunately, they arrive in your office frantic as they pull out two specimen cups, one with the patient's urine and the other with the tea and challenge you to distinguish them.

Recent URI is associated with IgA nephropathy

Tea colored urine, gross hematuria

How about that - they look identical! Instead of admitting this you ask for another specimen. The parents note that a similar thing happened 3 months ago, and the other doctor distinguished the two cups by tasting them, fortunately he picked the tea first. You pretend not to hear this as you

*(Continued on next page)*

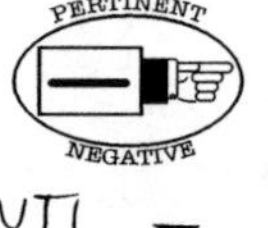


UTI unlikely

*(Continued from previous page)*

leave the room for an "emergency". There is no history of fever.

The patient has a low-grade fever. Blood pressure is 110/70 there is no rash, joint pain, edema or any other symptoms.

PUTTING NUMBERS INTO WORDS

Normal BP

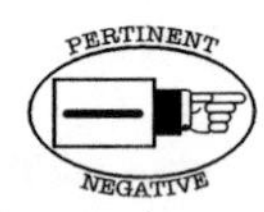


Protein losing nephropathy unlikely

The WBC is 9.5 with a normal differential. Electrolytes and serum complement levels are normal.

Limited to renal disease with normal complement levels

## Question 1:

C) IgA nephropathy

## Question 2:

D) Elevated IgA levels

## Question 3:

A) 10% chance of end stage renal disease

IgA nephropathy is more commonly seen in females and presents with hematuria often following a URI. It presents with microscopic or gross hematuria. Proteinuria may or may not be part of the presentation.

Serum complement levels are normal. The long-term prognosis in adults is worse than children. Up to 45% of adults progress to end stage renal disease whereas only 10% of children progress to this stage.

# Case 97

(see page 265 for Questions)

While playing outdoors with some friends a 7-year-old boy falls down and experiences a witnessed generalized tonic-clonic seizure. By objective accounts the seizure lasts a minute and a half. There was not trauma now nor in the past. Other than a documented febrile seizure at the age of 3 there is no significant neurological history, developmental delay or cognitive impairment.

An EEG done 2 days later demonstrates some left temporal slowing.

THE DIVERSION

The past history of a febrile seizure is not relevant

Witnessed generalized atraumatic seizure lasting 1.5 minutes

PERTINENT NEGATIVE

Left temporal slowing 2 days after the seizure is not relevant

 

## Question 1:

C) Non-urgent Head MRI

## Question 2:

D) There is a 1% greater chance of developing epilepsy than the general population

## Question 3:

D) EEG findings of spike discharges

While febrile seizures do not raise the chances of epilepsy developing *significantly*, there is a 1% higher chance of developing epilepsy than in the general population.

One generalized seizure in the absence of past neurological history, developmental delay or cognitive impairment would not justify starting anticonvulsant medication. It would not justify a stat head CT or MRI. However, obtaining a nonurgent MRI would be appropriate.

Left temporal slowing <u>2 days after the seizure</u> would not be a significant finding in deciding whether to start anticonvulsant therapy. However EEG findings of *spiked discharges* would be a significant finding in determining risk for future seizures and deciding whether to start anti-seizure medications.

# Case 98

(see page 269 for Questions)

One day after being bitten on the leg by her cat, the parents of a 6-year-old girl note increased swelling and tenderness at the site. Her immunizations are up to date and the cat has scratched and bitten her before so the parents are surprised at how red this has gotten so fast.

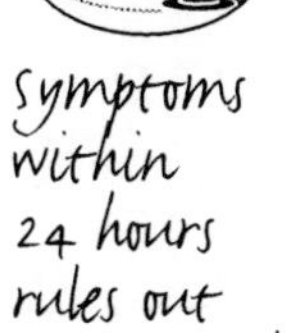


symptoms within 24 hours rules out cat scratch fever

## Question 1:

C) *Pasteurella multocida*

## Question 2:

B) Amoxicillin-clavulanate

## Question 3:

B) Ampicillin

A favorite board trick is to present you with a child who sustains a reaction to a cat bite or scratch hoping you would assume it is due to cat scratch fever. Even if you studied appropriately and realize that the infectious agent in cat scratch fever is *Bartonella henselae* you would actually be penalized anyway.

Cat scratch fever is a febrile illness that presents one-several weeks after the cat scratches (or bites – yes, we know it can also be transmitted after a bite – but the boards have to throw you some kind of bone!) In this case the symptoms came on within 24 hours and this is more consistent with an infection by *Pasteurella multocida*.

Effective antibiotics against *Pasteurella multocida* include:

- Amoxicillin clavulanate
- Penicillin
- Ampicillin
- Doxycycline
- Cefuroxime
- Cefpodoxime
- Quinolones
- Trimethoprim-sulfamethoxazole

 

However doxycycline and quinolones (such as levofloxacin) would be contraindicated in a 6-year-old patient when alternative medications are just as effective.

The following antibiotics are *not effective against Pasteurella multocida.*

- Dicloxacillin
- Erythromycin
- Clindamycin
- Cephalexin
- Cefadroxil
- Cefaclor

# Case 99

(see page 271 for Questions)

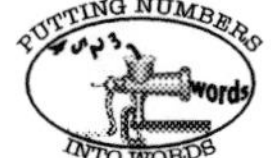


You are performing a routine physical examination on a full term newborn.

Micro-cephaly

On physical examination you note a head circumference of 30 cm with a purpuric rash on the legs and arms. The abdomen is soft with marked hepatosplenomegaly.

Purpura

Hepatosplenomegaly

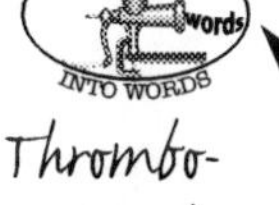


CBC reveals a white blood cell count of 9.5 with a normal differential and a platelet count of 85, hematocrit of 36 and a hemoglobin of 12. Bilirubin is 10.5/ 0.5

Thrombocytopenia

Hyperbilirubinemia

Ophthalmological consult confirms the presence of retinitis.

Chorioretinitis consistent with a diagnosis of congenital CMV infection

 

## Question 1:

D) Congenital CMV

## Question 2:

C) Periventricular cerebral calcifications

The combination of retinitis, hepatosplenomegaly, thrombocytopenia, purpuric rash and microcephaly points to a diagnosis of congenital CMV infection.

One would also expect to see periventricular cerebral calcification. Diffuse cerebral calcifications would be seen in congenital toxoplasmosis.

# Case 100

*(see page 273 for Questions)*

You are evaluating a 4-month-old infant for a routine well baby visit. The baby has been feeding well and is developmentally normal. The baby is sleeping while you are taking a history from the mother and you notice a jugular pulse wave. You auscultate the heart and hear a soft murmur which is consistent with a flow murmur and a resting heart rate of 60. You note that during previous physical exams the infant's heart rate is 80, 75, and 85.

*All findings while the baby is sleeping*

PUTTING NUMBERS INTO WORDS

*Bradycardia*

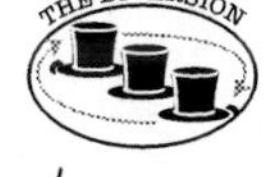


*These may have been measured while the baby was crying*

By now the baby has woken up and is crying because he is hungry. You listen to the heart rate again and it is 70.

*The heartrate increases with crying*

## Question 1:

D) EKG

## Question 2:

D) Congenital AV heart block

## Question 3:

D) Pacemaker

This patient presents with bradycardia at rest that increases with crying. This is consistent with a diagnosis of AV node heart block. The question is whether the previous higher heart rates were measured while the baby was asleep or awake. Since these heart rates are still low, and in all likelihood measured while the baby was asleep the correct diagnosis is probably congenital heart block, not acquired heart block.

The diagnosis would best be confirmed non-invasively via EKG.

Because of the risk for sudden death most infants with congenital AV block and bradycardia end up needing a pacemaker.

# Case 101

(see page 275 for Questions)

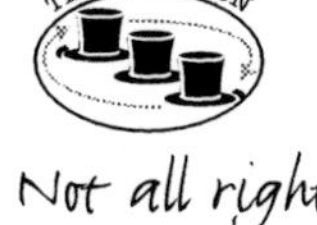


You are evaluating a 9-year-old girl with an acute onset of severe right-sided abdominal pain which is intermittent. She has been experiencing episodic vomiting. She has been afebrile with no diarrhea.

Not all right sided pain is appendicitis

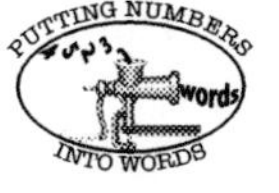


Normal WBC

CBC shows a WBC 12.5 with a normal differential, electrolytes are within normal limits. Urinalysis is negative for blood, bacteria, and protein. Abdominal x-ray demonstrates some stool on the left side with no signs of obstruction. Abdominal and pelvic ultrasound reveals an echogenic intraovarian mass.

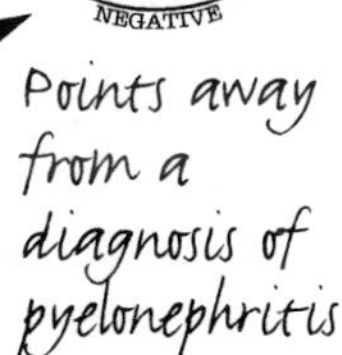


Points away from a diagnosis of pyelonephritis

Not enough evidence for constipation to explain presentation

Consistent with a diagnosis of ovarian torsion

## Question 1:

C) Doppler flow ultrasonography

## Question 2:

D) Ovarian Torsion

## Question 3:

E) Laparoscopic reversal of torsion

The presenting history and findings are most consistent with a diagnosis of ovarian torsion. The patient has *intermittent* pain which is severe with a normal white count and urinalysis. These point away from kidney stones, pyelonephritis or constipation.

If available, this can best be confirmed with Doppler ultrasound to assess ovarian blood flow. Once confirmed or even without confirmation if Doppler ultrasound is not available then laparoscopic intervention would be indicated.

 

# Case 102

(see page 277 for Questions)

Marked acute ataxia

You are evaluating a 7-year-old girl who has been having difficulty walking unassisted. On physical exam you note some weakness of the arms which is less pronounced than the muscle weakness of the lower extremities.

Ascending paralysis

The deep tendon reflexes are diminished in all 4 extremities. Sensory loss is limited to the face where you also note bilateral ptosis. There is no tenderness over the vertebral spine. The symptoms started late last night. Up until that point she has had no medical problems and her neurodevelopment has been normal and her immunizations are up to date.

ANSWER REVEALED

Consistent with a tick bite

Rules out transverse myelitis

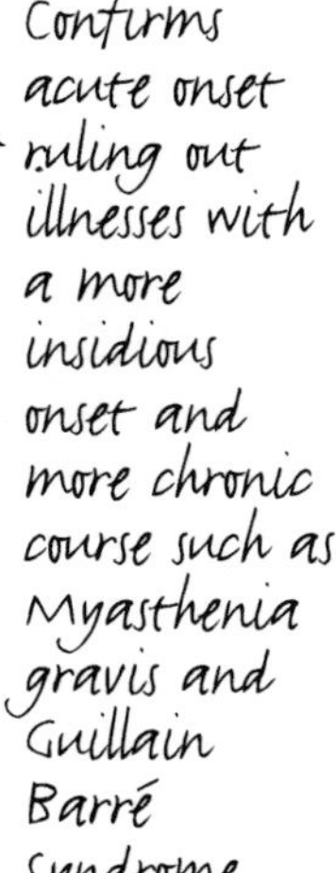
Confirms acute onset ruling out illnesses with a more insidious onset and more chronic course such as Myasthenia gravis and Guillain Barré Syndrome

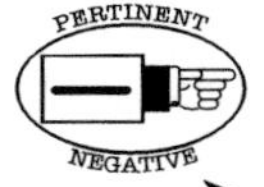
PERTINENT
NEGATIVE

## Question 1:

B) Tick bite

## Question 2:

E) Look for and remove all ticks

The patient is presenting with acute ataxia and symptoms consistent with a tick bite (neurotoxin) which includes sensory loss limited to the face, absence of deep tendon reflexes and ascending paralysis.

The onset within hours rules out more chronic illnesses or illnesses which present with a more insidious onset. The most appropriate management for the patient in this vignette would be to look for and remove all ticks.

# Case 103

(see page 279 for Questions)

You are evaluating a 3-month-old infant on a routine followup visit. The infant is a former 29-week preemie who was in the NICU for several weeks and required mechanical ventilation for around 10 days. He has been diagnosed with bronchopulmonary dysplasia and has been treated with furosemide. A routine urine dipstick is positive for blood.

Known to cause hypercalciuria which can cause microscopic hematuria

Not definitive for the presence of blood since it can also be positive for hemoglobin, myoglobin, and porphyrins

 

## Question 1:

B) Urinalysis

## Question 2:

C) Serum alkaline phosphatase

## Question 3:

A) Idiopathic hypercalciuria

A positive urine dipstick is insufficient to confirm the presence of RBCs in urine. This must be confirmed by Urinalysis, which would be the most appropriate next step in this patient.

Once the presence of RBCs in the urine is confirmed, the next step would be a spot urine creatinine: calcium ratio followed by 24-hour calcium quantification. Eventually it might be necessary to measure serum creatinine, calcium, and phosphate and urine calcium. It is unlikely that an alkaline phosphatase measurement will be needed.

The most common cause of microscopic hematuria in children is *idiopathic* which is Latin for "we haven't the foggiest idea!"

# Case 104

(see page 281 for Questions)

PERTINENT NEGATIVE

You are evaluating a 10-year-old girl who presents with a one-week history of crampy abdominal pain and malodorous diarrhea.

*Consistent with poor absorption*

She has not travelled outside of the U.S. over the past year and has not gone camping.

*Rules out amebiasis and giardiasis*

Her past history is negative except for a bout of pneumonia 6 weeks ago, which was successfully treated with a course of Azithromycin after a course of amoxicillin failed.

*Recent antibiotic treatment*

PERTINENT NEGATIVE

Physical examination is negative except for crampy abdominal pain.

*Negative for systemic symptoms*

She is in the 60th percentile for weight and height.

*Rules out chronic illness such as inflammatory bowel disease.*

Stool sample is positive for the presence of white blood cells.

*Consistent with colitis of any cause*

 

## Question 1:

E) Stool sample for the presence of Clostridium difficile toxin

## Question 2:

C) Pseudomembranous colitis

## Question 3:

A) Oral Metronidazole

The presence of WBC in the stool merely tells you that the patient has **colitis** but doesn't tell you much else. The fact that the patient did not travel recently rules out amebiasis and their specifically telling you that the patient did not go camping recently helps you rule out Giardiasis.

While most cases of pseudomembranous colitis caused by *C. difficile* toxin occur within 2 weeks of a course of antibiotics, it can occur within 10 weeks, as is the case in this patient. This makes for a diagnosis of pseudomembranous colitis caused by *C. difficile* toxin.

Therefore the most appropriate study would be stool sample for *C. difficile* toxin and the most appropriate treatment would be a course of oral metronidazole.

# Case 105

(see page 283 for Questions)

You are evaluating an 8-year-old girl who has fallen behind in reading. She seems to have difficulty reading both at home and in school.

Difficulty with reading specifically

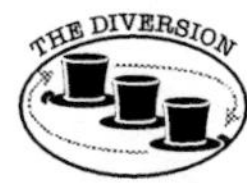


Commonly seen in children

You noticed her in the waiting room holding the magazine she was reading very close to her face. However the result of her vision check in your office is completely normal.

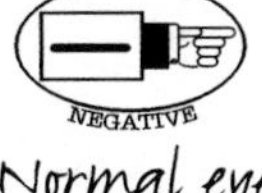


Normal eye exam

On physical exam her funduscopic exam is normal; pupils are equal and reactive to light. She sits in the front row where she is most comfortable and has no difficulty paying attention, gets along well with other children and is doing well in other subjects.

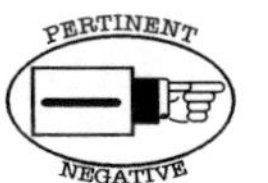


ADHD unlikely

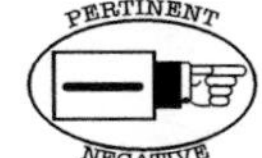


Points to a specific learning disability

## Question 1:

D) Specific learning disability

## Question 2:

D) Cognitive testing

## Question 3:

A) Myopia

The patient in this vignette has a specific difficulty and that is a difficulty in reading. Thrown in for good measure is noting that she holds the magazine close to her eyes. The 3rd question regarding the most common ophthalmological problem seen in children is additional fuel for the diversionary trail leading you to believe that the eyes are the underlying problem.

The problem is a specific difficulty with reading requiring cognitive testing to identify a specific learning disability.

By the way the most common ophthalmologic problem in children is myopia, which is nearsightedness (but you knew that).

 

# Case 106

(see page 285 for Questions)

You are evaluating a 3-year-old boy who has had a severe gastroenteritis for the past four days. Initially he was vomiting with watery diarrhea. Over the past day and a half the diarrhea has continued but he was able to hold down fluids and has been given water and apple juice which he has been tolerating well.

High risk for potassium loss

Slight risk for hyponatremia or hyperglycemia

PUTTING NUMBERS INTO WORDS

Despite this, he is lethargic with muscle aches, a heart rate of 115, respiratory rate of 25, and temperature of 100.3F. His capillary refill is less than 2 seconds, his mucous membranes are moist and he has good tear production.
His abdominal exam is benign with no guarding or rebound tenderness. He has urinated twice today.

Consistent with hypokalemia

Vital signs stable, low grade temperature

Clinical dehydration and/or sodium imbalance unlikely

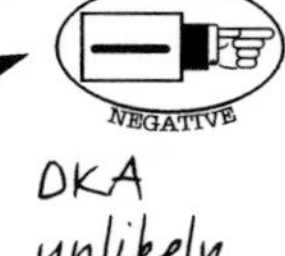


DKA unlikely

 

## Question 1:

A) Hypokalemia

## Question 2:

A) Life-threatening arrhythmias

## Question 3:

A) 12-lead EKG

This patient is presenting with gastroenteritis that initially presented with vomiting and diarrhea. The diarrhea has continued and the child is not showing significant clinical signs of dehydration or sodium derangement.

Although the free water could leave him at risk for hyponatremia (not hypernatremia) it is unlikely to be the cause of the problem. With diarrhea you have a direct ongoing loss of potassium.

This leaves the patient at risk for hypokalemia which would explain the fatigue and muscle aches. While you may be tempted to go straight to potassium replacement you must first identify if there are any cardiac arrhythmias present via 12-lead EKG which would be the most appropriate *initial* step you would take.

 

# Case 107

(see page 287 for Questions)

You are evaluating a 6-week-old male infant diagnosed with colic who now presents with large loose stools that contain bloody streaks. The mother initially breast fed for the first 4 weeks of life and started a standard infant formula upon returning to work.

Cow based formula heralds the onset of symptoms

On physical examination the infant is afebrile with normal vital signs. Abdomen is soft with normal bowel sounds.

PERTINENT NEGATIVE

Absence of systemic signs

The stool pH is 5.30.

Consistent with a diagnosis of cow milk protein intolerance

 

## Question 1:

D) Cow milk protein intolerance

## Question 2:

E) Protein hydrolysate formula

The infant developed signs of colitis with the onset of the use of cow based "standard" formula. There is no evidence of any systemic signs and symptoms one would expect with intussusception or an infectious etiology. In addition there is no evidence of galactosemia. Anal fissures would be more consistent with hard rather than loose stools.

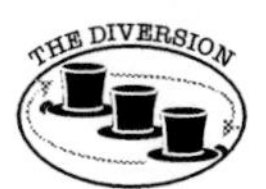


# Case 108

(see page 289 for Questions)

*Increased risk for cardiac disease but could be a red herring*

*Intermittent acrocyanosis*

A 6-month-old infant with Down syndrome is brought to you by his parents because of an intermittent history of episodes where his hands and feet turn blue. The rest of the time his hands and feet have a mottled appearance. He has been gaining weight steadily and on physical examination there is no murmur and the infant is not tachypneic nor in any distress while feeding. EKG is within normal limits for age and chest x-ray shows no cardiomegaly and normal pulmonary vascularity.

PERTINENT NEGATIVE

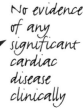

*A normal finding without cardiac disease*

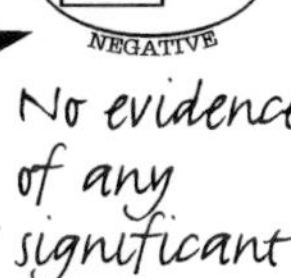


*No evidence of any significant cardiac disease clinically*

 

## Question 1:

B) Cardiac echo

## Question 2:

E) Cutis marmorata physiologica

## Question 3:

B) Decreased pulmonary vascular resistance

In this question the fact that the patient has Down syndrome is merely a diversion and makes it a trickier question on 2 fronts:

1) Children with Down syndrome are at increased risk for cardiac disease

 · Specifically ASD leading to a left to right shunt and ultimately resulting in Eisenmenger syndrome which is a result of irreversible pulmonary vascular disease.
 · This patient shows no signs of this.

2) All children with Down syndrome should have a screening cardiac echo – Therefore in this case a cardiac echo would be indicated.

THE DIVERSION

However this patient only has *episodic acrocyanosis* which results in mottling of the arms and legs in between episodes and this is called *cutis marmorata physiologica.*

*If this patient did not have Down syndrome then only reassurance would be indicated.*

Children with Down syndrome are at risk for

- Poor weight gain (with or without cardiac disease)
- ASD
- *<u>Increased</u> pulmonary vascular resistance*
- Left to right shunting
- Right ventricular hypertrophy

# Case 109

(see page 291 for Questions)

You are called to the delivery room to evaluate an infant who is apneic. The infant was delivered by elective repeat C/Section. There was no meconium staining. The delivery room staff has suctioned out the nasopharynx and found no meconium. They have been providing bag mask ventilation and you notice that the chest wall is not expanding and the infant appears to be cyanotic. You step in to take over the resuscitation.

Apneic full term newborn

PERTINENT NEGATIVE

Meconium aspiration and pulmonary hypertension very unlikely

Poor technique the likely cause

 

## Question 1:

A) Continue bag mask ventilation with increased pressures

## Question 2:

A) Transient tachypnea of the newborn

In this case the only definitive factor in the presenting history is inadequate chest movement during resuscitation. There is no evidence of congenital cardiac disease, meconium aspiration or pulmonary hypertension. While hyaline membrane disease or respiratory distress syndrome *can* occur in full term infants, there is nothing in the vignette to suggest this.

Infants born via C.-section are at increased risk for transient tachypnea of the new born which can result in initial apnea and/or respiratory distress. In this patient that is the most likely diagnosis.

# Case 110

(see page 293 for Questions)

Fine motor function deterioration

A 14-year-old boy has been experiencing difficulty holding objects in the morning especially when he has not gotten adequate sleep. He has similar difficulty holding other objects in the morning and occasionally has odd jerky movements of his arms that he cannot control. In the past he has been diagnosed with absence seizures but he is no longer receiving treatment. He has had no absence seizures for several years.

Myoclonic jerky movements

Past history of absence seizures

A recent EEG result shows bilateral 3 to 6 cycles per second polyspike and wave discharges.

Diagnostic for juvenile myoclonic epilepsy

 

## Question 1:

D) Juvenile myoclonic epilepsy

## Question 2:

B) Valproic acid

## Question 3:

A) 0%

Juvenile myoclonic epilepsy is commonly seen in the morning especially if the child is sleep-deprived. In addition a past history of absence seizures is sometimes seen.

An EEG with bilateral 3-6 cycles per second polyspike and wave discharges is diagnostic. The treatment of choice is valproic acid and they never spontaneously remit, requiring lifelong treatment.

# Case 111

(see page 295 for Questions)

You are evaluating a 10-year-old girl who has been experiencing intermittent diurnal urinary incontinence. She has previously been fully continent. She has been afebrile, experienced no dysuria, and is afebrile in your office.

Past medical history is completely benign

On physical exam there is no suprapubic tenderness and vaginal exam is unremarkable. Urinalysis is negative for blood, protein, leukocyte esterase and nitrites. Urine glucose is negative. A Urine culture grew out no organisms and spot urine revealed calcium: creatinine ratio of 0.12 (less than 0.2 is normal). She has otherwise been healthy with no prior illnesses or surgery.

UTI unlikely

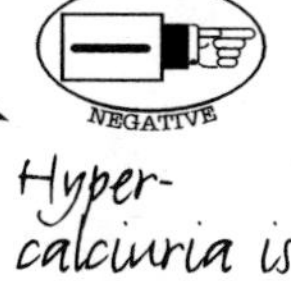


Hyper-calciuria is ruled out.

 

## Question 1:

A) Reassurance and management

## Question 2:

A) Unstable bladder

## Question 3:

A) Anticholinergic medication

The history and pertinent negative findings on history and physical in this patient is consistent with a diagnosis of *unstable bladder* (bladder dyssynergy) and at this point no further studies listed are appropriate other than reassurance. Unstable bladder is due to delayed neurological maturation of the micturition process. It is a cause of secondary diurnal enuresis. Anticholinergic medications can sometimes be helpful in managing this difficult situation until it subsides on its own.

 

# Case 112

(see page 297 for Questions)

You are evaluating an infant at his 2-week followup. The infant was born by normal spontaneous vaginal birth, and has done well up until recently when the mother noticed that he has been breathing fast and has decreased the frequency of and duration of feedings. In addition he appears to be sweating a lot.

Heart failure as the PDA closes

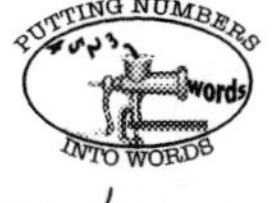


Tachypnea and respiratory distress

On physical examination you note that the baby is breathing greater than 75 per minute with nasal flaring. Peripheral pulses are weak especially in the lower extremity. On auscultation you note a gallop rhythm.

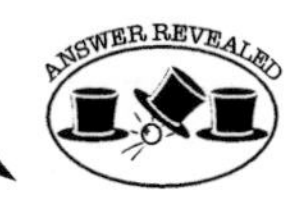


Points to a diagnosis of coarctation

## Question 1:

E) Coarctation of the aorta

## Question 2:

C) Cardiac Echo

## Question 3:

C) Prostaglandin E

The infant in the vignette is showing signs of congestive heart failure. The tachypnea is due in large part to pulmonary congestion due to diminished left heart outflow. This coupled with the diagnostic finding of diminished peripheral pulses, especially in the lower extremities, makes for a diagnosis of coarctation of the aorta.

This is best diagnosed with cardiac echo and the initial treatment would be prostaglandin E to maintain the PDA opened as much as possible.

The infant is acyanotic which all but rules out Tetralogy of Fallot and transposition of the great vessels. In addition, the history is inconsistent with these diagnoses.

# Case 113

(see page 299 for Questions)

A 2-year-old is brought to your office because of a peculiar rash brought to the parent's attention by the nurse at the day care center the child attends. The child is afebrile and other wise doing well with no prior history of pneumonia, recurrent otitis media or epistaxis.

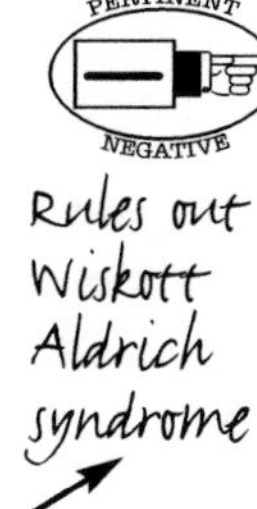


On physical examination the child is afebrile and you note a scaly rash on the scalp especially in front of the ears with a similar pattern in the underarms and diaper area. You note that the rash consists of several small lesions measuring 2-4 mm, which are erythematous brownish papules with some petechiae. Skin biopsy reveals monocyte macrophages containing Birbeck's granules.

Typical distribution for Langerhans cell histiocytosis or Class I histiocytosis

 

## Question 1:

A) Class I Histiocytosis

## Question 2:

C) Malignant histiocytosis

A scaly rash with erythematous brownish papules with some petechiae on the scalp distributed in the preauricular, axillary and diaper area is classic for Type I Histiocytosis. In addition, Birbeck's granules are pathognomonic.

To add to the confusion, Type I Histiocytosis used to be known as *Langerhans cell histiocytosis* and just plain old *histiocytosis X*.

*Birbeck granules* are pathognomonic for Type I histiocytoses and this category includes Hand Schüller-Christian disease, Eosinophilic granuloma, and Letter Siwe Disease. Once again, Langerhans Cell histiocytosis is the previous name for type I disease

Malignant histiocytosis would be under the category of Type III disease, where Birbeck's granules are not seen.

Histiocytosis can be confused with 3 other similar rashes and can be distinguished as follows:

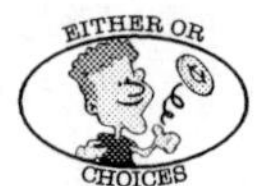


**Atopic Dermatitis** – Brown papules and petechiae are not seen and the diaper area is spared.

**Seborrheic Dermatitis** – Confluent salmon-pink scaling patches would be seen rather than discrete papules and petechiae as seen in this patient.

**Wiskott Aldrich syndrome** – they would have to include a history of recurrent infections and bleeding since thrombocytopenia is also part of the presentation. The rash would be consistent with atopic dermatitis as described on the previous page

 

# Case 114

(see page 301 for Questions)

You are evaluating a newborn at 2 weeks and note that there is difficulty with abduction of the hips. The gluteal folds, however, are symmetrical. You suspect bilateral subluxation on physical examination.

*This is an example of a vignette where they simply give you the diagnosis. Often this is done after wasting 10 minutes of your time reading the vignette; We decided to spare you the agony.*

## Question 1:

D) Ultrasound is diagnostic

## Question 2:

A) It is more common among females

## Question 3:

C) The Pavlik harness is the Standard treatment

Developmental dysplasia of the hip is not always evident at birth and the definitive diagnosis is made by ultrasound. However confirmation of treatment success is done by x-ray. Watch for the wording of the question.

The Pavlik harness is the standard treatment and double diapers are not considered to be reliable enough. The Pavlik harness must be done prior to 6 months, after that open surgical reduction is necessary.

Developmental dysplasia of the hip is more common among females, Caucasians and first-born newborns

Asymmetric gluteal folds may not be evident at 2 weeks. In addition, this finding (or lack thereof) is considered to be neither sensitive nor very specific.

# Case 115

(see page 303 for Questions)

You are evaluating an 8-month-old infant who has been distressed over the past 2 hours and unable to feed. You evaluate the infant and note that he is diaphoretic, pale and in significant distress and inconsolable. On physical examination the infant is afebrile with a respiratory rate of 50 breaths per minute but you have a difficult time obtaining a peripheral pulse. You place the infant on a monitor and note a heart rate of 250 with narrow complexes. Prior to this, the infant's growth and development were within normal limits.

Acute problem

Cardio-vascular compromise

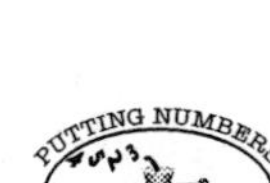


Tachypnea

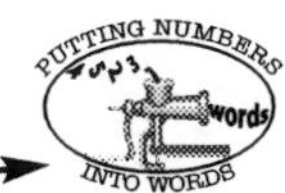


Tachycardia

Consistent with SVT

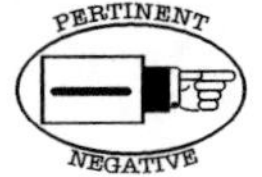


Rules out chronic problem

 

## Question 1:

E) Supraventricular tachycardia

## Question 2:

E) Adenosine IV rapid push followed by normal saline flush

This is an infant with a previous unremarkable history, ruling out any significant congenital heart disease. The combination of this and an acute onset of narrow complex tachycardia makes for a diagnosis of supraventricular tachycardia.

With an infant with SVT, cold compress or other vagal maneuvers should take second stage to *adenosine* via rapid infusion with a saline flush (since the half-life is extremely short).

This temporarily blocks the supraventricular impulse at the AV node level resulting in a "resetting" of the normal heart rate.

# Case 116

(see page 305 for Questions)

You are "taking a break" working as a camp doctor and you are holding your weekly clinic just before going bass fishing. A 12-year-old boy appears from *his* bass fishing trip wearing short pants and a tank top shirt. You, on the other hand, are wearing scrub cutoffs and a tank top lab coat despite the fact that your narcissistic lack of awareness is causing humiliating embarrassment for your children who are also attending the camp. He (we're back to the patient now) has gone fishing everyday for a week, and has developed a worsening rash over the past 2 days.

Areas of exposure match the distribution of the rash.

The rash appears on his arms and legs sparing his trunk, groin area, face and scalp. The rash is linear and pruritic with erythematous papules and vesicles.

Classic description of contact dermatitis, most likely poison ivy

 

## Question 1:

E) Contact Dermatitis

## Question 2:

D) Prednisone

## Question 3:

D) Type 4 allergic reaction

Despite the description of the child going fishing this is not ichthyosis. The description of the rash, the exposure to plants and the distribution of the rash over areas likely to come in contact with plants is classic for poison ivy contact dermatitis.

The area of distribution is greater than 15% of the body surface, which is why oral prednisone is the preferred treatment over topical corticosteroid.

Poison Ivy contact dermatitis would be a Type 4 or Type IV reaction.[2]

[2] As pointed out in *Laughing Your Way To Passing The Pediatric Boards®* this can be easily remembered using the mnemonic poison **IV** is a type **IV** reaction.

 

# Case 117

(see page 307 for Questions)

Abdominal pain, vomiting and bloody diarrhea

A 26-month-old boy in your practice presents with a history of vomiting and severe abdominal pain. In addition the parents have brought along a diaper containing bloody stools. The pain is severe and then will sometimes stop suddenly. He was seen in your office last week for an upper respiratory tract infection. The boy is afebrile

Pain is intermittent

Recent URI

He was initially sleeping and the parents asked that you hold off on examining him since he has not gotten much rest in the past 24 hours. You gently palpate the abdomen and note no tenderness, guarding or rebound.

They call you back into the room 15 minutes later. The child is now squirming and screaming in extreme pain. The abdomen is now tender with marked guarding. You are unable to assess for rebound tenderness due to the severity of the pain.

 

## Question 1:

E) Air contrast enema

## Question 2:

D) Intussusception

## Question 3:

D) Air contrast enema

This patient is presenting with intermittent abdominal pain with a calm asymptomatic period in between episodes. This points to a diagnosis of intussusception; in addition, intussusception is often preceded by a URI. There is not evidence of an infectious etiology or inflammatory bowel disease.

# Case 118

(see page 309 for Questions)

You are evaluating a 12-year-old boy who, up until this point, has been healthy, in fact, quite athletic. He presents this morning with weakness of the entire left side of his body. His cognition and speech are within normal limits as are his hearing and vision.

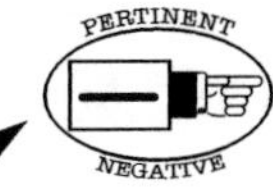


Left sided hemiplegia

On physical exam you note marked motor weakness of his left lower and upper extremities and marked tenderness over his chest where you note ecchymoses. The patient then recalls getting hit in the chest by a rushing opponent yesterday who knocked the wind out of the patient but he was able to finish the game. There was no loss of consciousness and he denies getting hit on the head at all.

Seemingly innocuous but the likely explanation of the presentation

Makes subdural, epidural hematoma and basilar skull fracture unlikely

## Question 1:

D) Carotid angiography

## Question 2:

E) Embolic stroke

In this case the incidental finding of ecchymoses and the additional history regarding the blunt chest trauma are the key to the answer. In this case, the blunt chest trauma most likely caused carotid dissection resulting in a thrombus forming, which then embolized. .

This is why *carotid angiography* would be the best study to identify the source of the problem and the cause of the presentation would be an embolic stroke resulting in the left hemiplegia.

# Case 119

(see page 311 for Questions)

You are evaluating a 14-year-old boy brought in by EMS to the pediatric ER. He was found passed out in the back yard by his friends. You are unable to arouse him although he does respond to painful stimuli. His pupils are miotic but equal and reactive. His temperature is 97.8 F; respiratory rate is 10 with a shallow breathing pattern. His heart rate is 55 and blood pressure is 95/65.

Comatose

Pinpoint pupils

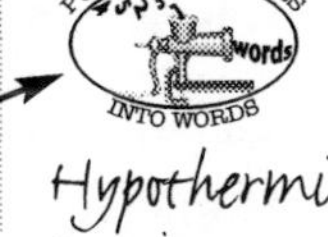


Hypothermia
Respiratory depression
Hypotensive

 

## Question 1:

D) Opiate overdose

## Question 2:

D) Endotracheal intubation

## Question 3:

D) IM naloxone

The combination of pinpoint pupils (miosis), hypothermia, bradycardia, hypotension and shallow breathing make the most likely diagnosis opiate overdose.

Anytime you are presented with a comatose patient, regardless of the underlying etiology you must follow the ABC's of CPR. In this case priority is with protecting the airway and the most appropriate immediate step to take in this patient is endotracheal intubation.

Once the patient is stabilized it would be appropriate to then administer naloxone, which is an opiate antagonist. It would serve the dual purpose of reversing the opiate toxicity and establishing a correct diagnosis.

# Case 120

(see page 313 for Questions)

You are evaluating a 15-month-old boy who has been vomiting for 48 hours with copious watery diarrhea. He has had no wet diapers today. On physical exam the toddler is very ill appearing and listless, with a temperature of 101.2, heart rate of 180. Abdominal exam is remarkable for doughy skin with no guarding or rebound tenderness. Capillary refill is greater than 3 seconds.

Marked decreased urine output

Consistent with severe hyper-natremic dehydration

PUTTING NUMBERS INTO WORDS

Febrile, marked tachycardia

Severe dehydration

## Question 1:

B) Severe

## Question 2:

B) Hypernatremic

This patient is clearly dehydrated. Regarding the degree of dehydration and type of dehydration one has to look at signs in the history and physical to determine this.

The doughy skin substantiates the diagnosis of hypernatremic dehydration.

Capillary refill greater than 3 seconds along with a "very ill appearing child" who is "listless" is consistent with severe dehydration.

Since hypernatremic dehydration is usually a result of intracellular dehydration with the preservation of extracellular fluid volume, clinical signs of dehydration usually occur late in the game making the significant signs in this patient even more concerning.

# Case 121

(see page 315 for Questions)

An 18-month-old child in your practice has been observed by his parents and baby-sitter eating dirt on numerous occasions. His growth and development are normal. His immunizations are up to date and his height and weight are at the 60th percentile for age. His nutrition is appropriate for age.

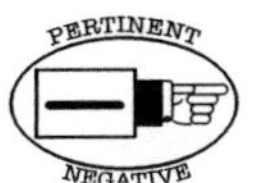


Rules out Visceral larva migrans

On physical examination the child is afebrile, TMs intact, funduscopic exam is unremarkable. His abdomen is soft with hepatosplenomegaly.

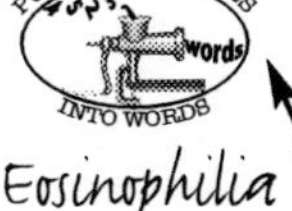


Eosinophilia

His screening CBC shows a WBC of 12.5. Hematocrit is 38 with hemoglobin of 12.5, 10% neutrophils 10 % lymphocytes and 80% eosinophils, platelet count of 175.

 

## Question 1:

C) Toxocara canis

## Question 2:

D) Serological testing

## Question 3:

B) Albendazole

A child who has a history of eating dirt and presents with eosinophilia has a parasitic illness. In the absence of hepatosplenomegaly, fever, or ophthalmological findings a diagnosis of visceral larva migrans is all but ruled out. There are no signs of plumbism or lead poisoning on CBC. There are also no clinical signs consistent with Enterobius vermicularis.

Toxocara canis is diagnosed by serological testing for antibodies and is treated with albendazole or mebendazole.

# Case 122

(see page 317 for Questions)

You are assigned a full-term newborn born to a 35-year-old multigravida recent immigrant from Guatemala. The infant had an indirect bilirubin level of 12.1 and direct of 0.4 at 6 hours of age, which is now 19.4/0.4—the baby has had stool production

Greater than 10 prior to 24 hours, not physiologic

Consider something which is routinely treated and monitored for in US, i.e. RhoGAM administration

Requires phototherapy

The mother is O negative and the baby is B positive. The infant on exam is icteric with a soft abdomen, no hepatomegaly. Heart S1, S2 no murmur, with normal retinal exam with good red reflex. The baby is alert and responsive. Other than mild cephalohematoma the baby is normocephalic with no abnormalities noted.

Points away from TORCH diseases

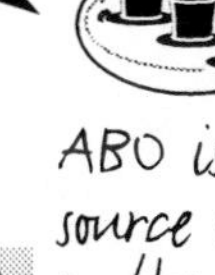


ABO is not the source of the problem, the Rh factor is more likely. Mom is Rh negative, baby positive, which is a set up, especially since she is a multip.

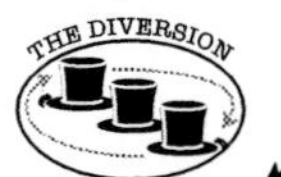


Diversion to lead you to believe that hemolysis is the cause of the problem

 

## Question 1:

E) Rh incompatibility

## Question 2:

D) Phototherapy and hydration

This mother is from another country, which on the boards often means she did not receive treatment she might have received in the US. Therefore since she is Rh negative one would expect her to have received RhoGAM. However if she did not this would explain the infant developing hyperbilirubinemia within 24 hours, which by definition is not physiologic.

Therefore Rh incompatibility is the likely explanation requiring phototherapy.

# Case 123

(see page 319 for Questions)

A 16-year-old girl presents with an erythematous rash on her cheeks and nasal area. In addition she has a rash on her hands which is also erythematous, scaly and limited to the dorsal aspect of her hands in between the joints. The patient has been experiencing thinning hair and hair loss. On physical examination the patient experiences sharp chest pain with inspiration.

Malar rash

scaling thick plaques between the joints – SLE

Alopecia common in SLE

 

## Question 1:

B) Serum Antibody to SM nuclear antigen

## Question 2:

A) False positive VDRL

The patient in the vignette has SLE. Therefore the best way to diagnose this is via Serum Antibody to SM nuclear antigen... SLE is associated with false positive VDRL, not FTA-ABS

Dermatomyositis is associated with proximal muscle weakness and positive Gower's maneuvers.

The rash that appears on the dorsum of the hand in dermatomyositis and SLE can be very similar. If you are presented with a picture or it is described watch for the subtle differences.

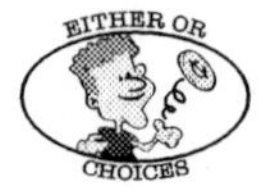


| | SLE | Dermatomyositis |
|---|---|---|
| Rash on Hand | Dorsum of the hands- knuckles are *not involved.* Described as scaling thick plaques | Gottron's papules, lesions are flat topped, erythematous *involving the knuckles* |
| Rash on Face | Involves cheeks and nose, in a "malar", "butterfly" distribution | *Violaceous rash involving cheeks and eyelids* described as *heliotropic* |

SLE is between the knuckles. SL**E** is betw**ee**n the knuckles

Dermatomy-**o**-sitis is **o**n the knuckles

# Case 124

(see page 321 for Questions)

A 12-year-old boy presents with a circular violaceous rash which, when palpated, feels like there are firm papules underneath.

Classic description of granuloma annulare

He was treated with topical nystatin for 10 days followed by a ten-day course of clotrimazole with no clinical improvement.

PERTINENT NEGATIVE

Rules out tinea corporis

## Question 1:

E) Granuloma annulare

## Question 2:

E) Reassurance that this will resolve spontaneously

The rash described is classic for granuloma annulare for which there is no treatment other than reassurance that it will spontaneously remit.

# Case 125

(see page 323 for Questions)

THE DIVERSION

You are evaluating a 16-year-old girl with a 7 week history of mild anxiety and increased heart rate evaluated at the local ER and dismissed as pre exam jitters with a normal EKG; she has lost 7 pounds in the past month. You ask her about her weight and she tells you that she is okay with it but is concerned about the weight she lost.

Clearly not the correct diagnosis

Unlikely to be an eating disorder

On physical exam she is afebrile, somewhat anxious but appropriate. Her heart rate is 110 with a respiratory rate of 18 and blood pressure of 135/85. Cap refill is less than 2 seconds with 2 + pulses throughout. You note a soft systolic ejection murmur heard best on the left side. Her abdomen is soft with no hepatomegaly. Lungs are clear. EKG reveals a sinus tachycardia with a normal p wave preceding each QRS complex of normal width.

Not likely to be an anxiety attack

PUTTING NUMBERS INTO WORDS

Tachycardia, normal respiratory rate, mild hypertension

No mention of a delta wave – Wolf Parkinson White ruled out.
Normal QRS width – SVT ruled out

 

## Question 1:

D) Hyperthyroidism

## Question 2:

B) Thyroid Stimulation hormone level

The history and findings in this patient are consistent with hyperthyroidism. The patient is mildly anxious, with tachycardia, mild hypertension and weight loss that is troubling to the patient. An anxiety or eating disorder is unlikely in this case.

The EKG findings are inconsistent with Wolf Parkinson White and SVT. Therefore, the next most logical step would be to obtain a thyroid stimulating hormone level (TSH).

# Case 126

(see page 325 for Questions)

You are evaluating a 5-month-old infant who, up until 3 weeks ago, was growing normally and doing fine. Over the past few weeks he has become increasingly tachypneic and has not gained any weight. Physical exam reveals a respiratory rate of 75 and grade 2 systolic ejection murmur with no signs of cyanosis. The EKG is normal and the chest x-ray reveals increased vascularity with no cardiomegaly.

A disorder which manifests after the neonatal period requiring time to develop

Signs of heart failure and failure to thrive

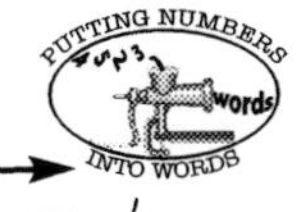


Tachypnea

PERTINENT NEGATIVE

Rules out cyanotic heart disease

Right sided overload

## Question 1:

E) Supracardiac total anomalous venous return

## Question 2:

D) Increased right-sided pre-load

Supracardiac total anomalous venous return results in the pulmonary vein returning oxygenated blood to the right side through the left inominate and vertical veins leading to the superior vena cava.

This results in *right sided overload* leading to

Mixing of deoxygenated blood into systemic circulation via foramen ovale

Pulmonary congestion

If sufficient mixing occurs cyanosis may not be present. However, pulmonary congestion results in *tachypnea and pulmonary edema worsening during the first weeks to months of life resulting in failure to thrive.*

# Case 127

(see page 327 for Questions)

Typical distribution of psoriasis

A 6-year-old presents with a rash that has developed over the past two months. The rash is seen on the extensor surface of the knees, they eyebrows and behind the ears. On physical exam you note erythematous raised plaques. On the extensor surface of the elbows you note pinpoint areas of hemorrhaging.

Typical description of psoriatic rash

Auspitz sign

 

## Question 1:

B) Psoriasis

## Question 2:

C) Topical steroids

## Question 3:

E) Koebner phenomenon

The description, distribution and inclusion of Auspitz sign make the diagnosis of psoriasis straightforward. Psoriasis is best treated initially with topical steroid creams and it is associated with **Koebner phenomenon** which is the appearance of lesions in areas of scratches and abrasions.

Psoriasis can be confused with *nummular eczema* but can be distinguished:

EITHER OR CHOICES

**Nummular eczema** – presents with oozing crusting erosions and/or macules with fine scales. *They are not raised.*

# Case 128

(see page 329 for Questions)

A 2-year-old boy presents with a recurrent rash that is best described as scaling patches which are erythematous and concentrated on the upper and lower extremities, face and the scalp with sparing of the diaper area.

Typical description of Atopic dermatitis

The boy has been hospitalized 3 times for lobar pneumonia; during one episode blood cultures grew out *Streptococcus pneumoniae*. He also has experienced recurrent epistaxis.

Recurrent infection, pneumococcus, and epistaxis with a history of atopic dermatitis

On CBC he has a WBC of 12.5 with a normal differential. Hematocrit is 38 and his platelet count is 40 thousand.

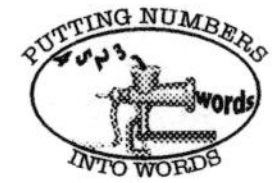


Thrombocytopenia

 

## Question 1:

E) Wiskott Aldrich Syndrome

## Question 2:

C) Atopic dermatitis

## Question 3:

C) X- Linked recessive

There are 3 components of Wiskott Aldrich syndrome present in this vignette, which should make it an easy 3 questions to answer correctly.

Those 3 components are:

1) Recurrent infection
2) Thrombocytopenia
3) Atopic dermatitis.

Atopic dermatitis is present in patients with Wiskott Aldrich syndrome, which is inherited in an X-linked recessive pattern.

MNEMONIC This is easily remembered by changing the spelling to WiXkott Aldrich syndrome.

# Case 129

(see page 331 for Questions)

A 4-year-old girl returns from a trip to Long Island to visit her grandparents and presents with fever, muscles aches, shaking chills and headache.
Three days later you note a petechial rash on the wrists and ankles.
Her immunizations are up to date.

Rocky mountain spotted fever is endemic there

Classic presentation of Rocky Mountain spotted fever

Measles ruled out[1]

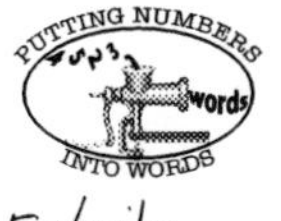


On physical exam the child is low in energy and cranky and has a temperature of 102.

Febrile

[1] On the boards, not in real life. As of the writing of this book, there is a widely publicized measles outbreak.

 

## Question 1:

C) Rocky Mountain spotted fever

## Question 2:

E) Implement treatment only

## Question 3:

A) Doxycycline

This patient is presenting with a classic history for Rocky Mountain spotted fever caused by *Rickettsia rickettsii.* They will never present a patient just returning from the Rocky Mountains, that would be too easy. Long Island is a more typical location on the boards.

Treatment is with Doxycycline, even in children younger than 8 since the risk for teeth staining isn't as much as a concern as inadequate treatment. When Rocky Mountain spotted fever is suspected there is not time for testing, implementation of treatment should be started right away.

 

# Case 130

(see page 333 for Questions)

You are caring for a 15-year-old boy who presents with severe headache, runny nose, sore throat and a temperature of 101.2 F. A cough that started 3 days ago has gotten much worse to the point that his voice is hoarse. Auscultation of his chest is significant for rales and wheezes throughout the lung fields. You order a chest x-ray that reveals bilateral interstitial infiltrates concentrated in the lower lobes.

Consistent with strep or mycoplasma

Consistent with mycoplasma pneumonia

All of his immunizations are up to date and he has not done any recent travel.

Makes pertussis unlikely

 

## Question 1:

A) Serological testing for Mycoplasma pneumoniae

## Question 2:

D) Mycoplasma pneumonia

## Question 3:

E) Azithromycin

This patient is presenting with classic signs of mycoplasma pneumonia. The best way to test for this is via measuring mycoplasma titers.

Cold hemagglutinins will only be positive in 50% of cases and would not be the best method to make the diagnosis. The treatment of choice would be azithromycin.

# Case 131

(see page 335 for Questions)

Multifocal clonic seizure activity confirmed

You are evaluating a newborn on day two of life who has been experiencing clonic seizures which have been observed independently by 3 nurses. You have been called to observe an episode which you note lasting 120 seconds involving the hands and left leg. The Apgars were 8 and 9 and the delivery was a spontaneous vaginal delivery although vacuum extraction was required. The CBC and electrolytes are within normal limits. Bilirubin 1/0.5 total and direct.

High risk for subarachnoid hemorrhage

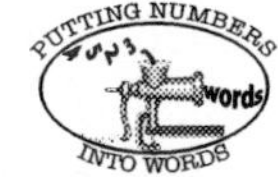

A lumbar puncture is done with the following results:

Marked xanthochromia with RBC 1200/cubic millimeter
Protein 600 mg/dL

Bloody atraumatic tap with elevated protein, consistent with subarachnoid hemorrhage not meningitis

## Question 1:

C) Head CT

## Question 2:

C) Subarachnoid hemorrhage

## Question 3:

C) Serial head circumference evaluation

The combination of a vacuum extraction delivery and a presumed atraumatic grossly bloody lumbar puncture with elevated protein and xanthochromia would suggest a subarachnoid hemorrhage not meningitis. Hyperbilirubinemia is not a factor. There is no evidence to suggest herpes encephalitis either.

The best study to confirm this would be a head CT and management would be watchful waiting, including serial head circumference measurements.

# Case 132

(see page 337 for Questions)

You are evaluating a newborn who has had wheezing present since birth. The wheezing is worse whenever the child is feeding or crying. The mother also notes that the wheezing gets worse whenever the infant's neck is flexed. A right-sided aortic arch is noted on chest x-ray.

Congenital

Wheezing worse with crying, feeding and neck flexion

Suggests vascular anomaly.

 

## Question 1:

C) Vascular ring

## Question 2:

C) Barium Swallow

A wheeze since birth is by definition congenital. The x-ray of a right-sided aortic arch suggests an anatomical-vascular etiology. Wheezing which worsens while crying, feeding, and especially with neck flexion would suggest a vascular ring, specifically a double aortic arch in this case. A barium swallow would be the most appropriate study to help solidify the diagnosis.

# Case 133

(see page 339 for Questions)

A 2-1/2 year old toddler was found with an opened bottle of his grandmother's imipramine pills. They are not sure how many pills were in the bottle and there were some contents found on the toddler's mouth and tongue. On physical exam the toddler is alert and responsive, afebrile and vital signs stable.

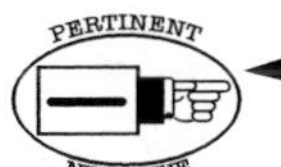


Not much to figure out here, they are essentially telling you the child ingested imipramine and they are testing your knowledge on managing the case

 

## Question 1:

E) Miosis

## Question 2:

C) Activated charcoal

## Question 3:

C) Baseline EKG

When taking care of a child who ingested imipramine the initial steps should be to reduce absorption. This is best done via activated charcoal *without sorbitol.* In a toddler the inclusion of sorbitol would increase the risk for severe dehydration and subsequent electrolyte imbalance. Imipramine can also result in cardiac arrest. Mydriasis would be a sign of imipramine toxicity, *not miosis.*

Imipramine ingestion can result in *hyper*tension initially and *hypo*tension later on. The primary concern is for dangerous arrhythmias and therefore EKG monitoring would be the most helpful in monitoring this patient.

 

# Case 134

(see page 341 for Questions)

You are evaluating a 2-day-old newborn who presents with bilateral leukocoria and routine hearing screening suggests sensorineural hearing loss. You also note facial purpura lesions and hepatosplenomegaly.

Absent red reflex

Associated with congenital rubella

Blueberry muffin rash

## Question 1:

A) Congenital rubella

## Question 2:

A) Pulmonary artery stenosis

An infant with sensorineural hearing loss, blueberry muffin rash and leukocoria would lead you to a diagnosis of congenital rubella which is also associated with pulmonary artery stenosis.

# Case 135

(see page 343 for Questions)

You are evaluating a 3-year-old child with a chronic rash described as dry, scaly patches concentrated on the extensor surfaces and the face since infancy. He now presents with oozing crusting lesions that are not scaly as previous lesions were and are not responding to previous treatments which, in the past, have been successful.

Atopic Dermatitis

Secondarily infected

## Question 1:

B) Bullous impetigo

## Question 2:

B) Oral Antibiotics

This vignette describes a child with atopic dermatitis since birth which is now crusted and oozing and not responding to usual treatments. This would be classic for chronic atopic dermatitis that is secondarily infected resulting in bullous impetigo requiring oral antibiotics.